"The greatest medical discovery of our time is the power within the human body to heal and rejuvenate itself. This tremendous discovery is destined to change the way we practice medicine in America. In the future, instead of cutting the body—instead of drugging it, instead of working against its natural systems, doctors will strive to feed and enhance the body's amazing power to self-heal.

The medical establishment still seems to believe that nutrition cannot prevent disease, and is practically useless in treating it. Yet, we now have scientific proof that diet is the single most powerful tool for the treatment of disease. More powerful than drugs. More powerful than surgery. More powerful than anything in the doctor's bag.

And you can do it yourself. The medical profession is too narrow minded to admit the enormous value of nutritional healing."

Dr. JULIAN WHITAKER, M.D.
WHITAKER WELLNESS INSTITUTE, NEWPORT BEACH, CA

Published by: Genetic Press Longmont, CO

First Edition: March, 2006

Printed by: Inland Books

Cover Design by: Desert Dolphin (www.DesertDolphin.com)

Library of Congress Cataloging-in-Publication Data
Ohlgren, Scott, 1956–
Tomasulo, Joann, 1959–

The 28 Day Cleansing Program

$28.00

ISBN: 0-9721483-4-5

THE 28-DAY CLEANSING PROGRAM

The proven recipe system for skin & digestive repair.

SCOTT OHLGREN & JOANN TOMASULO

www.HowHealthWorks.com

Contents

PART TWO: RECIPES   85

PART THREE: SAMPLE 28 DAYS OF RECIPES
AND CLEANSING TIPS   179

"Every life form on the planet survives in a specific environment. Change the environment and you automatically change the species which resides in that habitat. As you will never see a giraffe in the arctic, nor a penguin in the tropics, you will also never see the normal friendly microorganisms that we were meant to have in an acid bowel. Nor will we see pathogenic bacterial, yeast, and parasites in a clean healthy body."

DR. RICHARD ANDERSON, ND

PREFACE

REAL STORIES,
REAL SOLUTIONS

2

*I was walking through a Seattle health food store and I saw this book, called **Cellular Cleansing Made Easy.** Its title screamed out at me. I am a 48-year old professional woman that has struggled for decades with low energy, weight gain, depression, allergies, dry skin, and moments of memory lapses. I decided to do Scott's program.*

I had many challenges with this cleanse. It was a radical lifestyle change to the way I had been living. Even though I did not do everything Scott talks about, I did what I could do and stayed focused on it every day.

When I look back, I am amazed at what I accomplished in those 28 days. People need to hear these results:

- *I no longer have depression. I am happy, and deal with life's daily challenges.*
- *I no longer have sinus headaches (a minor miracle).*
- *My skin is beautiful! No longer dry, do not need lotions and does not itch!*
- *No more constipation or bloated feeling.*
- *I lost 17 pounds.*
- *I am off of the 3 prescriptions I was on for depression, allergies and thyroid.*

Thank you for opening my eyes, freeing me from the medicated fog, and helping me live a better life.

SHELLY CLEATOR
EVERETT WASHINGTON

Before doing the cleanse, I was depressed and tired all the time. My left knee and shoulder were constantly in pain. I did the program outlined on Scott's 28-day system, and much to my surprise, the pain in both joints disappeared. Who would have thought that these were, in any way, connected to my food choices? Better still, my depression has left, and my mind is so much clearer. No more pills and medication. Thank you for a healthier body and mind.

ELIZABETH BLACKBURN

A year ago at age 46 I began experiencing tiredness and an unusual blistering and extreme itching of the skin of my fingers. I couldn't sleep, the pain was so intense at times. I visited a dermatologist who spent one minute with me, and then wrote out a prescription for both topical and oral steroids. At my wits end, I dutifully and foolishly filled the prescriptions. When the last dose was used, the condition returned, worse than before. I knew that there must be a cause, and that I needed to find it, and not just cover it up with drugs. Exasperated, I researched online for any hope, and found Scott Ohlgren's website. I read all the articles and participated in his online chat board, where he graciously answered my questions personally. I purchased his CD/book program, and went shopping for new foods, cookbooks and supplements to take care of my own condition. After a few days of initial detoxification (which he had warned about) and feeling very tired, I began to feel better... look better... and my fingers showed improvement within a week. After a month on the regime, my condition was completely gone, as were a few unwanted pounds and under-eye circles.

It has been a year since that awful experience. My skin now has a new softness and smoothness, and I have so much energy again. The real surprise, a true bonus, is that I have a new, more joyful outlook on life.

The information Scott shared in his 28-Day Regeneration Program allowed me to participate in my own healing, and I am a loyal fan. Blessings!

GINGER NARMOUR

Rosacea runs in my family and I'd been plagued with it for several years. The traditional creams and gels were only moderately effective. When I started Scott's cellular cleansing program, I was not particularly thinking about it improving the rosacea.

What a pleasant surprise to find that within a couple of weeks, my Rosacea was completely cleared up. In fact, whenever it reappears has become my gauge for knowing that it's time to do some internal cleansing, just as Scott's program taught me. Thank you for these skills.

KATHRYN LINVILLE

By the time I found this cleansing program, I had a growing list of ailments, including Irritable Bowel Syndrome so bad that I had to go many times during the day. I had headaches almost constantly. My skin was so oily that my makeup would not stay on longer than 2 hours, and I would constantly have to wipe my face off with a tissue. I also had a mild depression going on. I would worry about my health and really felt powerless to do anything about it.

I heard about your program and knew immediately that I had to try it. As soon as I started, I realized it was something I could actually do, that it wouldn't be hard. Soon I was juicing, and colon cleansing, and sweating, and eating delicious healthy foods. I began to see the connection between these symptoms and what I had been eating. The results were amazing:

Within three weeks, I noticed not only was I not depressed, I was exhilarated and felt like dancing in my kitchen. As a matter of fact, I did dance. Some other changes:

- I completely got off of the antidepressant medication. I have had moments of feeling truly ecstatic.
- I started having normal bowel movements. I can not tell you how that freed me up to go about a normal schedule during the day.
- My skin cleared up and became much less oily. I don't even get oily hair after half a day.
- My Irritable Bowel Syndrome completely went away.
- No more headaches!
- I no longer depressed; I honestly had never felt better in my life.

It is now been 9 months. I will not give up this healthy lifestyle. I refuse to ever go back to eating the way I used to eat. I will be eternally grateful for what you and your website have done for me.

BARBARA ALLEN

I suffered toxic heavy metal exposure from 9/11 in NYC, which then became disabling the next year when we rented a home that was inundated with black mold. After that, I knew that I had to detoxify my body in order to begin the process of healing. But trying to undo 35 years of my previous eating and lifestyle habits proved near impossible, especially on my own.

After attending one of Scott's live seminars, I read his book and embarked on a journey that would be the beginning of a new life. My boyfriend and I did the 28-day cleanse together (which actually helped us grow even closer), and within weeks, I could feel my body shifting.

Because of the intensity of my toxic overload, I wasn't a candidate for a miraculous, immediate healing, but the cellular cleanse Scott provided showed me a clear and easy path that has allowed me to permanently change the way I eat and even think about food. This new mindfulness, in turn, has given my body the opportunity to do what it wants to do—heal itself.

After the 28-day jump start, I've continued with the lessons I learned from the book and CDs, and over time my gut has healed, my brain fog has cleared, my chemical sensitivities lessened, my hair stopped falling out, my skin cleared up, and I have a much more positive outlook. Most of all, I can actually see the light of recovery. My boyfriend, who was not suffering from toxic injury, also experienced improved energy, mood, and clear skin. We both still follow the cleansing protocols (foods, sauna, colon care, skin brushing) in our daily lives.

JILL SVERDLOVE
BOULDER, CO

I hate to speak of something so personal, but I feel that it is so important for other women to know about. I am now 44, and in the midst of menopause. When it started, I was sluggish, gaining a lot of weight (over 30 pounds), and my sex drive had driven away. I heard about Scott's book, and did my first cleanse in May, 2005. The first week, my digestive system kicked in, I could actually feel it.. The second week, I felt charged with energy and the third week, my sex drive pulled up in front of the house. By the forth week, I had lost 12 pounds and established some new habits.

I feel women in this stage of life can truly keep their metabolism going, and hardly feel the symptoms of menopause. I am so sincerely pleased.

CAROLYN G
MCKEAN, PENNSYLVANIA

6

I found Scott's book while searching for a way to improve my health. At 43 years old, I have survived 4 teenagers, cancer, thyroidectomy, a spine rebuild, rheumatoid arthritis, and McDonalds. I have followed the program for almost 5 months now. My biggest win is that I have removed 8 daily prescriptions.

I don't do this program perfectly at all. Yet the progress is unbelievable. I hope that's an inspiration to others, because you can get results without being perfect. JUST DO IT.

And my students have commented frequently, "boy you are happy today!" And you know I am! Thanks, Scott, truly!

SANDY SCOTT

As a professional adventure racer, I'm always looking for a way to improve performance. Last year, my boyfriend convinced me to read Cellular Cleansing Made Easy. I thought it would be easy, since I didn't smoke, drink caffeine and work out five to seven days every week. Was I ever in for a surprise.

One evening during the first week, I started choking up some phlegm. My boyfriend grabbed (I'm not kidding) a bucket and I started spitting out all this gunk. It was draining out of my nose and throat and lungs. I spit up clear goo for about an hour and a half. My boyfriend, who had done other cleanses, was elated. He told me all about detoxification and explained that my body was ridding itself of toxins. I immediately shared my story on Scott's online forum.

Around the 10th day, I started seeing unexpected results. I felt clearer; my brain seemed less foggy. I started doing some of the physical transformers outlined in the book, like saunas, skin brushing, and colon care. A few weeks in, a friend and I cheated and went out for pizza. We both felt so heavy, mucus-laden, and constipated the next day. What a lesson!

The end results: I have never felt so sharp or light or good. I am regular now for the first time in my life. My skin has a glow it didn't have before, and friends actually comment on it. I lost 17 pounds that I didn't need; and a problematic knee no longer hurts when I run and bike. Although my diet is not pristine, I have become very aware of what I put in my body now. I know what's right for it and what's wrong. I have lent out the 2 copies of the book to numerous friends who have each done the cleansing program. Thanks for everything Scott, you changed my life.

MICHELLE LYMAN, ADVENTURE RACER

I found that this cleanse not only changed my views on food, but other people's views of me as well. I look healthier, and people often tell me that I'm glowing. I have a much more consistent positive outlook—no more emotional sugar roller coasters.

What Scott talks about is a common sense that has been lost to a world of convenience. But once people actually see the results that internal, cellular cleansing provides, they start to realize how food impacts health.

To those considering doing their first cleanse: rest assured you will feel these results, too. You will naturally begin to apply aspects of what you learned during your cleanse to your everyday life, because falling back into your old habits just seems so unappealing. The basic wisdoms you will obtain are well worth a little extra time and effort. I recommend that everyone does this.

Thanks, Scott.

JOSEPHINE MARTORANA

I have struggled with acne since the age of 15, and within the initial week of Scott's program, I realized my face was clearing up—for the first time in over 20 years. What a powerful, powerful message. Here I had tried almost every acne medication available (as an MD, I had access to them all), and yet within a week, I realized that Scott was dealing with the true cause of the why acne and other skin problems happen in the first place.

With acne in particular, the role of a clean colon became obvious; a clean, well-working colon also had a nice side benefit: it took about 5 pounds off, and gave me a trimmer waist.

Scott's detoxifying methods have also made a big difference in my mental clarity and all-around energy. I feel better than I have felt in a long time.

Since I have experienced the healing power outlined in Scott's program, I now pass this knowledge on to my patients. What we eat has a profound effect on our health. I knew this in my mind before my cleanse, but now I know it in my body and spirit.

Thank you for this amazing, life-changing experience.

DR. KRISTIN, MD
MEMBER, AMERICAN ACADEMY OF FAMILY PHYSICIANS

"As a nation we have come to believe that medicine and medical technology can solve our major health problems. The role of such important factors as diet in cancer and heart disease has long been obscured by the emphasis on the conquest of these diseases through the miracles of modern medicine. Treatment—not prevention—has been the order of the day.

The problem can never be solved merely by more and more medical care. Our greatest bulwark against the interests that have helped to create the present problems is an informed public."

DR. PHILIP LEE, PROFESSOR OF SOCIAL MEDICINE
AND DIRECTOR OF THE HEALTH POLICY PROGRAM
UNIVERSITY OF CALIFORNIA, SAN FRANCISCO

Part One

Understanding Cleansing
&
Getting Prepared

Acid Reflux, Acne, Allergies, Barrett's Esophagus,
Biliary Tract Diseases, Bloating, Boils, Candida,
Celiac Disease, Cholecystitis, Chronic Belching, Chronic Gas,
Colitis, Colon Cancer, Constipation, Crohn's Disease,
Cysts, Dandruff, Dermatitis,
Dermatofibroma, Diarrhea, Diverticulitis,
Dry Skin, Duodenal Ulcer, Eczema, Endometriosis,
Exocrine Pancreatic Insufficiency, Intestinal Dysbiosis,
Intestinal Permeability,
Fatty Liver, Fecal Incontinence,
Fibromyalgia, Folliculitis,
Gallstones, Gastritis,
Gastro-Esophageal-Reflux Disease,
Gastroparesis, GERD, GI infections, Heartburn,
Hemorrhoids, Hernia, Hiatal Hernia,
IBD, IBS, Indigestion, Inflammatory Bowel Disease,
Irritable Bowel Syndrome, Kidney stones, Leaky Gut Syndrome,
Malabsorption Syndrome, Peptic Ulcer,
Pimples, Proctitis, Psoriasis,
Rosacea,
Ulcerative Colitis...

CHAPTER 1

Our current reality

Take a quick look over at the facing page. The list of symptoms is alphabetical for easy viewing.

If you live in a western culture, chances are good that you suffer from one of these symptoms.

Chances are even better that you know someone who suffers from one or more of these symptoms.

But the highest odds— almost 100%—are that you have been taught the following:

Number 1: these symptoms have little to do with what you eat;

Number 2: the best way—the only way, really—to get rid of these symptoms is through pharmaceutical drugs; and

Number 3: if there is no cure yet, it will be forthcoming, once a few billion more dollars is spent in drug research. We just need more research money, and another drug to put into your bloodstream. Once that is accomplished, you will be cured.

What you have been taught is not true. Every one of those symptoms, from Rosacea to Crohn's to IBS, is there because of the internal condition your current diet has created. More importantly, every single one of those skin and digestive and allergic injuries can be healed, completely, through little else than a cleaner choice of food.

In case you glossed over that last sentence, let's restate it, because it is the central theme of this book: **a change to a clean nutritional intake can eliminate all of these symptoms.**

If you don't believe that, I don't blame you. Thirty years ago, I was entrenched in the same health model that we're talking about here, the one most of us have come to view as truth. Essentially, it is a belief that says *"these health problems have little to do with your lifestyle, and even less to do with your food choices. Just keep eating whatever you've been eating, because your symptoms did not appear on account of your diet, and they certainly won't disappear by a change in diet. That's just silly, because these symptoms are diseases, and you can't reverse that through food."*

> *"The greatest part of all chronic disease is created by the suppression of acute disease by drug poisoning."*
>
> Dr. Henry Lindlahr, M.D.

Armed with this belief system, I found myself at the age of sixteen, dutifully taking a pill—called tetracycline—twice a day, waiting for the next pharmaceutical acne cure that I knew was just around the corner. Every now and again, I would ask my dermatologist in Waukesha, Wisconsin, "Are you sure my skin problem has nothing to do with my food choices?" He would give me that "don't be silly" look, and explain that his entire profession had ascertained that skin problems were the result of a complex process that had nothing to do with diet. He would then hand me another three month prescription of tetracycline, and I would go back to eating my daily normal food choices. I say "normal," because it was what I was fed growing up, and because everyone around me ate this way. This included boxed cold cereal, pasteurized cow milk, luncheon meats, mayonnaise, Tang, Pop-Tarts, Twinkies, Hostess Ding Dongs, Spam, Rice a Roni, Swanson TV dinners, SpaghettiOs, Kraft Singles and Velveeta cheese, candy bars, McDonalds, ice cream, Welch's grape juice, hydrogenated oil and margarine, canned meat, canned fruit and canned vegetables. There were many other weekly ingredients, but remember, *none of it mattered*, since the world's top skin specialists were betting their reputation on the certainty that acne and other skin problems had little to do with someone's daily food choices.

Ask anyone who has ever used antibiotics for skin problems, and they will tell you that the problem never goes away. Neither did mine, even though I continued using that powerful drug every day, twice a day, for just over four years.

Finally, at the age of 20, a friend who was a student of natural health pointed to my face and said, *"That will go away if you stop eating that,"* pointing to my baloney, mayonnaise, and white-bread sandwich. She then explained how to do something called a nutritional cleansing program, where I would exchange my sludge-producing diet for what she called "cleansing" foods—foods closer to their whole, original form.

Within five weeks of starting the program, my acne was gone. Within two months, a growing sinus problem completely disappeared.

I knew right away that what my friend had shown me was not just about acne. It was about something much deeper, and about health problems far beyond my face.

From that first cleansing program, I was hooked. I learned everything I could on the diet/disease, diet/symptom connection. In the pre-Internet 1970s, this meant searching around for hard-to-find books, like Dr. Weston Price's *Nutrition and Physical Degeneration* (originally published in 1939), and anything from authors like Bernard Jensen and George Ohsawa.

As with any new field of study, you start to uncover a network of students, teachers and practitioners who have followed a thread of inquiry that often goes back many years. In this case, I learned that this diet-symptom/diet-disease connection was not some new revelation, something just discovered. In fact, there was a thread that could be traced back to Hippocrates (*"Let food be thy medicine, and medicine be thy food"*) and beyond.

It was an odd cast of characters, those of us following this natural food, natural healing thread, ranging from hippies to Nebraskan housewives, to a few MDs trying to remain anonymous, to registered dieticians no longer able to live with the methods and message of their profession, and to young guys like me, just trying to figure out how to stay healthy. While at first glance there seemed to be no commonality among us, there was often one shared experience: we had all rescued ourselves from a health challenge. We had each changed what we were eating, and lost a set of symptoms in the process. The other common theme was that we didn't want a diet. We wanted a health plan for our lives.

That first cleanse occurred in 1976. Bar none, periodic cellular cleansing has been the single biggest reason why I have stayed drug free, pain free, and symptom free for the past 30 years. After practicing the food/health connection, becoming a teacher and lecturer on the topic, and selling over 60,000 books, tapes, and videos on health, **here is what I know for certain: the large majority of every digestive problem, skin condition, allergy,**

heart condition, blood/ bacteria/ fungus/ yeast/ internal terrain mess is the result of a metabolic toxic overload, stemming directly from the life-deadening and historically new food chain we and our children are currently consuming. Any witness to this healing process can no longer conclude that Crohn's and Proctitis and allergies and eczema are not diseases that just happen, but instead are each the end, visual result of a nutritional toxic process that started a long time ago, and are as close to home as hand to mouth.

By reading this book, you are entering this same knowledge base that threads back for centuries. And as you start to apply this knowledge to your daily life, here are some of the things you will discover:

— Those of us living in western cultures are eating a diet that is historically new. At no other time, since the birth of humankind, have humans chosen to eat what we are eating. We are doing a giant nutritional experiment, and it is not working.

— Our food choices are constantly affecting our internal environment. Change this environment, and your symptoms will change.

— Real food can repair a diseased state.

— Most diseases should be viewed as an system-wide "ecological" problem, not a disease problem.

— There is no complex trick to healing. It's like getting in shape: you just need to work at it a bit every day.

— Your diet is the very first thing to look at once you start getting symptoms. Everything else is secondary.

— You can get rid your skin or digestive problem in the next month or two.

— Many allergies are caused by a clogged up digestive tract and liver. Clean them up, and your allergies can disappear.

THE GOOD NEWS & THE BAD NEWS

The good news is that you don't even have to believe in the diet/disease, diet/symptom connection—that your skin or digestive disorder is connected to your current food choices. This is because your body will prove it to yourself by following this 28-day program. It will become self-evident.

The bad news is that you are going to have to stop eating the way you've been eating, and learn to eat a healing, cleansing diet. There is no other way. You can not dance around this one particular requirement. Nutrition is the foundation on which everything else is built. While other modalities can be crucial—even life-saving—to your health, a change in what you feed your cells, at every meal and every snack, is the biggest imperative. You simply can not eat the same diet and expect to heal your symptoms by adding other modalities—even the ones that Joann and I advocate here.

This is hard news for some people to hear. Eating can be one of the most emotionally-based actions we humans do each day, and because of this, messing with your food can mess with your emotions. Yet if you are interested in getting rid of that symptom that has hounded you for years, there is no way around it: you have to start eating as if your digestion, your skin, and the loss of your allergies depended on it.

After years of teaching the diet/disease, diet/symptom connection, I find at this point, people fall into two distinct categories: those that are ready to just jump in and start, and those that can't quite believe that this is true; that their current set of symptoms can actually be reversed by simply changing what they're eating.

For those that belong to the first group: turn to the section that describes the 28-day program outlined in this book. Just do it. In a few short weeks, you'll be emailing us in elation, describing all the changes your body is going through.

For those that belong to the second group, I would suggest a couple things.

The first would be to read this entire book, from beginning to end, just to get used to its ideas. Next, realize that this idea that better food choices can reverse a disease is no longer considered a wacky idea. It is now well accepted that dietary changes can enable diabetics to get off their medication. Heart diseases can be reversed through a change in diet. Breast cancer is related to hormones in the blood, which are determined by the foods we choose each day. Kidney stones can be prevented—actually, dissolved— by a stopping certain foods, and adding others.

Next, pick up a copy of *Cellular Cleansing Made Easy*, as well as the 3-CD audiobook, *Real Food, Real Health: How to eat our way back to a health nation* (both can be found at www.HowHealthWorks.com). These will introduce you to more ideas on how the food/symptom connection works, and why. Also visit our online forum, to hear from some of the people with success stories who post there.

"The person who takes medicine must recover twice, once from the disease and once from the medicine."

Dr. William Osler, M.D.

CHAPTER 2

Why bother?

W̲e are a funny culture. We acknowledge the importance of daily body hygiene: we clean our skin, our hair, our teeth. But we are very blind to the parts of our body that we can't see.

Think about it: most of us know that brushing our teeth is an important part of staying healthy; we have figured out that by gently scrubbing our teeth, even carefully cleaning between each one, our mouth and teeth stay clear of health problems. We have also figured out that daily showering is a good thing for the health of our skin. We further know that it is important to wipe crumbs off the counter, to wash our dishes, and to wash our clothes on a regular basis.

DAILY INTERNAL HYGIENE

Yet we have no acknowledgement—we don't teach it in school—of the importance of doing a similar cleaning up of our internal organs, like the liver, the gall bladder, the large and small intestines, or the kidneys.

In terms of living a life free from disease, this is a very big oversight. Clogged up and toxin-filled organs are the main reason for the breakdown of physical health, and it doesn't take a whole lot of extrapolation to see that they are the main reason behind out-of-control health care costs.

Look at the following section on our internal organs (as well as the images

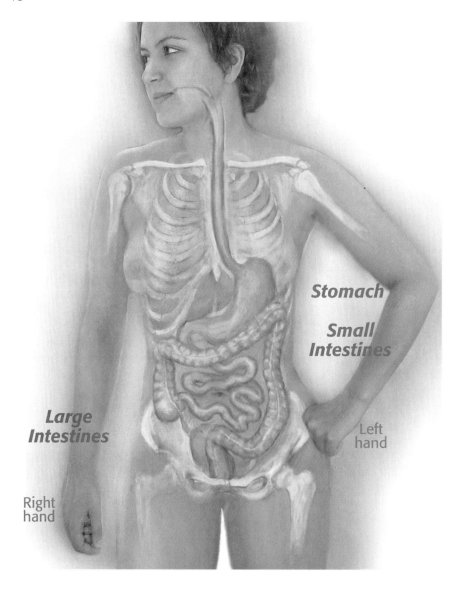

Stomach

Small
Intestines

Large
Intestines

Left
hand

Right
hand

commissioned from Dr. Nina Ollikainen, M.D., one of the finest present-day anatomical artists). You will start to get a sense of the far-reaching effects that malfunctioning organs have on our health. External hygiene like daily showering and hair grooming is good, but they pale in comparison and importance to internal hygiene. Let's look at why cleansing might be a good idea.

Your colon needs cleansing

After 20 years of teaching cleansing principals, I am now starting to see friends go under the knife from digestive auto-poisoning problems. Some of them have died. None of those good friends ever gave their digestion system any thought. For years, I could not figure out why they didn't treat their colon like they treated their hair, skin or teeth.

I now believe that one of the reasons for this blind behavior is this: we are a culture deeply embarrassed by basic human biology. We're embarrassed by bowel movements, to the point where we now have millions of people pooping once or twice a week, thinking that is enough, and normal, never wondering why we have the world's highest percentage of colon disease. We are a culture that thinks flushing out the colon with pure water is weird and unnatural, yet it is considered polite and normal and good logic for someone to walk into a building (called a hospital), be knocked unconscious, have their belly slit open with a sharp knife, and have twelve feet of intestines removed because that section has become necrotic and poisoned. People who go to colon hydro-therapists are considered "really out there," yet we live in a culture that considers it normal to spend $14,000 (*"Don't worry, it's covered by my health insurance, so no one is actually paying for it."*) to have a half-inch flexible hose/light/video camera and cutting instrument placed five feet up in through the anus in order to remove balls of toxic fleshy material protruding into the intestinal wall. And where high school kids are regularly taking drugs for uncontrollable diarrhea, and where over 80,000 American adults are now daily wearing adult diapers.

Our colons need our help and our attention. A cleansing diet helps strengthen peristaltic action, so the contents move along more regularly. Real food helps create the internal environment where friendly bacteria thrive and Candida and yeast and fungus have a hard time surviving.

Your kidneys need cleansing

Have any doubt? Just ask the 300,000 Americans currently on dialysis machines. Then look at the other 80,000 that need to walk around with adult diapers each day, and just over 1 million suffering and bleeding from kidney stones. Each one of these statistics speak about one thing: kidneys that have

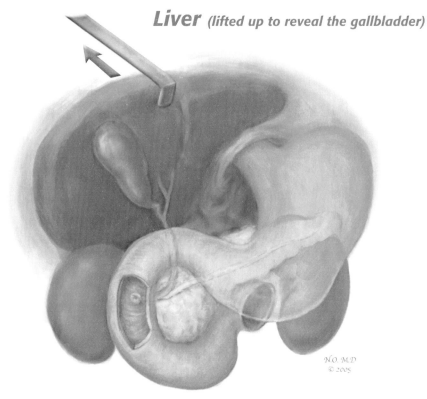

Liver *(lifted up to reveal the gallbladder)*

N.O. M.D
© 2005

Kidneys

lost their ability to function. This loss of function is often self-created, and can be self-corrected.

Although not often acknowledged in the West, kidney health has a close connection to sexual health. They also help regulate the chemical composition of blood, and play a role in hormones. A little known fact: about one and a half quarts of blood pass through the kidneys each minute. What's in our blood must pass through the kidneys. When the kidney's filtration system gets blocked, the body can no longer get rid of waste products, and these build up in the body. This buildup of metabolic waste results in uremia: literally, urine in the blood. According to western medical texts, symptoms associated with this backed up waste include headache, nausea, vomiting, poor appetite, extreme fatigue and mental cloudiness. From the eastern viewpoint, kidney problems can show up as excessive fear, anxiety, sexual insecurity, fear of letting go, and being chronically "pissed" off.

Again: we acknowledge the importance of cleansing our teeth and skin... why not our internal organs, like the kidneys?

YOUR LIVER NEEDS CLEANSING

Oh boy, does it ever. Our largest and most complex organ, the liver is responsible for over 600 different tasks. Look at the following short list, and think about the larger effects of each one:

— The liver filters and cleans about two quarts of blood *every minute.*

— It removes the large majority of the body's waste products, including absorbed plastics, smog, drugs, alcohol, skin creams, etc.

— Each day, it produces up to a quart of bile, the body's ultimate fat breakdown juice.

— The liver breaks down hormones, playing a vital role in our endocrine system, as well as our emotions.

— It stores extra vitamins, minerals, glucose, and even extra blood.

— It plays a major roll in our energy levels, our emotional levels, and is the key organ to getting rid of allergies.

And that is just the start. According to Western medical texts, symptoms associated with liver problems include bad breath, abdominal bloating, poor digestion, headaches, moodiness, coated tongue, sluggish metabolism, a weakened immune system, excessive body heat, menstruation problems, sugar cravings, and many others. Both Multiple Sclerosis and ALS (Amyotrophic Lateral Sclerosis, or Lou Gehrig's Disease) have been associated with severe liver dysfunction.

From the Eastern viewpoint, liver problems can show up as short temper, frustration, trouble falling asleep, inappropriate strong anger and rage, trouble with decision making, irritability and bitterness. Clearing out the liver/bile ducts is considered by some health professionals to be the most powerful procedure that you can do to improve your health.

I believe that the next big advance in understanding health will be in acknowledging the importance of self-detoxifying and de-sludging our liver. True, if you look into any human biology book, it already tells us that there are now over 600 known functions of the liver. But what we don't realize is how that functionality is dependent on how unclogged it is.

I can't say this enough: **a cleansed liver is a felt sensation**. Improving its function seems to affect everything, from mental clarity and focus, to emotions, to sleep, to how stress is handled, our digestion, our skin, even how we perceive and deal with—at least in my experience—relationships.

There are so many other reasons for doing a cleansing diet. Weight loss, joint pain, regaining sexual function, pre- and post-diabetic symptoms, better brain function... the list is endless. Cleansing repairs the body deeply, and gives it a chance to operate at a higher level of function.

The good news is that a cleansing diet has a cleansing effect on all of our organs. What we eat directly changes the quality of our blood. Our blood is then carried to the every cell of our organs. Clean blood makes for unclogged, fully functional organs.

It's not hard

People ask all the time: is cleansing, like, *hard*? My response is always the same: What is hard is living with symptoms. What is hard is living with a self-created, slightly diseased body. *That* is hard. That is downright difficult.

Cleansing is not hard. As a matter of fact, we've been doing it all our lives. We are cleansing right now, and have been since the moment of conception. Every one of our 100 trillion cells is constantly peeing and pooping, constantly taking in nutrients and getting rid of the old and used up, and has been doing this since that first cell division while in utero. Every time we breathe out, we've cleansed our body of the metabolic waste known as carbon dioxide. Every time we have a bowel movement, our body is eliminating old cellular material (interesting: up to 40% of every bowel movement is not our last few meals, but dead cells being sluffed off from all over the body). Cleansing occurs because our body's cells are constantly dying and being replaced with new cells. Our spleen and liver and stomach cells do it, our intestinal walls do it, even our bones and muscle cells do this regeneration circle of life. **All a cleansing program does is intensify the results.**

If you are not happy with the level of your health, you need to learn the art of building your fundamental biology. Just as a master gardener learns to build strong soil, impervious to blight and bugs, we can do the same and learn to build strong blood. **Strong blood means strong immunity.**

We know that if we pollute our external environment—the air, the water, the soil—then that which lives off those things is sickened. We need to extend that same awareness to our internal environment, our internal terrain. If what we are eating is not creating a healthy bloodstream, then this sea of nutrients that we float in, and are fed by, will not support vibrant health. We get symptoms.

It is now time that our culture acknowledges the role that a cleansing diet and lifestyle can play in eradicating many of these problems we are suffering from. It is learning how to build and repair our own biology, something that should have been taught in grade school. But it's never too late: you can start now, today, regardless of your age.

In most cases, impaired health is more the result of indulgences and practices that are absolutely harmful, than it is the result of omissions. Most sick people are very anxious to find out what they can do to get them well. What they fail to ask is, 'What can I stop doing that is making me sick?'

Dr. Ralph Cinque, M.D.

CHAPTER 3

How to use this book

The idea for this book came from the thousands of readers who read *Cellular Cleansing Made Easy*, and listened to the 3-CD audiobook, *Real Food, Real Health: how to eat our way back to a healthy nation.* These together made up the *28-Day Regeneration Program* I created in order to explain the power of nutritional cleansing. While the book and CDs laid out the how-tos of doing cellular cleansing over a 28-day period, it purposely didn't have many recipes. It instead suggested the foods to eat and not eat, and left readers to figure out their meal plan on their own.

However, many readers emailed us and said that they really wanted a much more exact daily regimen to follow—recipes to use for each meal, exact ways of setting up their kitchen so that it produced healing food easily, as well as the best tools for doing that. Some actually said that without that kind of stricter guidance, they know they wouldn't complete the program.

After thinking about it, I realized that I related to this request for a more exact daily structure. I had examples in my own life, in which someone's exact guidance made all the difference between procrastinating and not getting the results, and actually doing it and getting great results. For example, I would not have shown up faithfully at my gym every week for the past five years if it weren't for Sam Iannetta, my personal trainer at Functional Fitness USA, who not only holds me accountable, but also tells me precisely what to do each visit (*"Do this exercise, three times. Now do this one."*). He shows me what to do to get the results I'm looking for, and also creates the environment that makes me want to hold myself to a higher standard, to do what I know is good for me. He also creates the humor: *"Uh, are you pausing for a reason?"*

This accountability is what this book is about. It is designed to act as your personal trainer for each day of the cleansing program. I chose my long-time friend, Joann Tomasulo, as co-author, who worked tirelessly for two years cataloguing her best-tasting recipes that fit a cleansing program. And as you will see, days one through twenty-eight each have their own two-page spread, clearly marking the day's meal suggestions and other actions. We chose a book design that lays flat for easy use in the kitchen. There is even an important section on how to create and stock a pantry designed for health.

While *The Real Food, Real Health Book* is designed to work as a stand-alone book, you may find it helpful to review the original *Regeneration Program* (the book and CDs). However, you can use just this book to successfully experience and follow the cleansing program outlined here.

DIFFERENT WAYS, BUT NO EXCUSE

In my own experience dealing with life's entropic challenges, all of my best achievements have come about by setting up a game plan in advance. In other words, making the decision that from *this* date, to *this* date, I will do these XYZ daily actions. With this simple "put it in my calendar" trick, I have found that there is

> *"THINK. PLAN. DO. FINISH.*
> *I've yet to find a better method for breaking a bad habit and creating a new one. I repeat these four words over and over whenever I find myself stuck in a rut.."*
>
> SCOTT

no better way to create a new habit, or break an old one. **By setting up a future start and stop date**, you are able to override many of the aspects of inertia. You already do this in many other areas of your life. For example, work: you have to be there by 8 AM, or you get fired; and you can go home at 5 PM. Or with travel: you have to be at the airport on a certain date at a certain time, or you'll miss the connection; same with coming back. When I decided to run my first 26.2-mile marathon (I wasn't even jogging at the time), I hired a coach who said that the first step to completing that goal was to find a marathon race happening about four months into the future, *and register for it.* I did, and the effect on any inertia I had about training was immediate. I went out and bought a pair of running shoes, printed up a training schedule and taped it to my refrigerator and front door. I started training the next day. I successfully ran that marathon four months later.

So, the only rule that I would suggest for using this book would be to "put it on the calendar." Look over the program and decide on a 28-day period.

However, we don't all live the same lifestyle. We don't all live in the same weather climate, have the same daily demands, or marital and child status, or same budgetary and time restraints. So there are a variety of ways to feed yourself during your cleanse:

—**Follow the book exactly.** Prepare your kitchen as described. Purchase all the kitchen tools. Do the meal plan precisely as suggested, making every single delicious menu. Prepare for the following day's meals. Cook and make every meal yourself, in your own kitchen.

—**Follow the book roughly.** Use the recipes as a guide, but mix and match throughout the days' suggestions.

—**Do the cleanse with someone else.** Share cooking and preparation with a neighbor or friend across town. Think gym buddy, but for internal health.

—**Hire a part-time cook 5-10 hours/week.** Before you laugh that off as a silly idea that you can't afford, think again. You would be amazed at the number of talented young folks who not only know how to cook cleansing meals, but would love the chance to do it for what they currently earn working at the mall. I know this from firsthand experience: my wife and I have used part-time personal cooks in our home every week for over 10 years.

—**Graze at the deli** of your local food co-op, Whole Foods, Wild Oats, Earth Fare, Garner's, Mrs. Gooch's, Vitamin Cottage, or whatever health food store you live near. If you are too busy to juice and eat well, you are not too busy to stop at the store.

The point is this: there is no good excuse for not doing a cleansing program. You can not use lack of time, lack of resources, or any thing else as a valid reason for getting yourself off the prescription drug merry-go-round. Where there's a will, there's a way. It is time to treat nutrition as one of the most important aspects of your life.

MAKE IT EASY

Whatever method for cleansing you decide to use, one rule applies: you have to make it easy. If you make it hard to get healthy, you will not follow through. So, here are the 3 factors you must put into place:

1. **Organize your kitchen into a cleansing one** (see the Pantry section for this)

2. **Choose a definitive start and stop date.** Joann and I have outlined a 28-day program. So decide which day you will start and, 28 days later, which day you will finish. Put in on the calendar.

3. **Prepare your food chain.** Think about where you normally get your food and snacks during the course of a day. Think about where you get hungry. You need to be ready in those places with snacks and meals that lie inside of a cleansing diet instead of going down to the candy machine at work, or stopping at the convenience store while getting gas.

Purchase pre-made foods when possible. For instance, we show you how to make your own garbanzo bean hummus and your own juice. If you don't have the time, pick these prepared foods up at the health food store.

Learn the art of leftovers. If a recipe calls for rice, make enough to add to the next morning's cereal, or for lunch the next day. If you end up with some prepared food, will it work in the next soup? If tomorrow calls for beans, soak them the night before. Slow-cook your morning cereals over night, so you wake up with breakfast prepared. Think ahead.

Use other sources. Some recipes from your other cookbooks will fall into the guidelines of a cleansing program. Don't be afraid to use them.

AVOID THE FOOD WARS

As soon as anyone starts talking about a particular food choice, a large majority of the population rolls their eyes, and for good reason. Food has become politicized, and even religious-ized.

There are numerous food philosophies that describe how to best stay healthy. They run the entire gamut, from the Mainly Protein diets, to Only Raw Foods, to Absolutely No Animal Protein, to the Grain-based Theory, to Traditional American, Traditional European, and Traditional Ancient. And everything in between. They have names such as vegetarianism, macrobiotics, vegan, traditional, Atkins, Ayurvedic, and many others.

As you start seeing the deeper role that your food choices play in whether you get symptoms or not, and whether you get sick or get healthy, a personal food philosophy or preference is a natural conclusion to come to. However, creating a religion around it is not. There is a very big difference between seeing what works for you and being dogmatic.

I want to make a suggestion: the world has reached its limits of dogmatic thinking. It really doesn't need any more. It is not necessary to join a food group in order to understand the power of nutrition. You don't need to declare allegiance in order to get healthier.

> *"Don't be trapped by dogma, which is living with the results of other people's thinking."*
>
> STEVE JOBS
> CEO APPLE AND PIXAR

Joann and I are not promoting any one school of food politics in this book. Instead, we are teaching you the energetics of food. How food works in your body. One only needs to study a bit of dietary epidemiological history to see that there are many diets that can work to keep humans healthy and living drug free well into old age.

One of my passions and reasons for doing this work is to point out that there is more than one way to cleanse, and more than one way to stay healthy. Therefore, having some flexibility in your food beliefs and diet is not only necessary, it can be liberating, adventurous, and help keep you sane.

In the end, I do not really care how people experience becoming symptom-free. I only care that they learn that their diseases are largely self-created. And cleansing is a critical key to returning to pure health.

It is only human to pick up beliefs about health and food and diet as we move through life. My suggestion is this: ask yourself on a regular basis, *"Is what I believe about food and health true? Who told me, who influenced my decisions? Is it still true for them? Is it still true for me?"*

Examine your beliefs about food yearly, just as you look at other factors that contribute to the quality of your life. You are not the same person you were five years ago. You may need completely different fuel today.

WHAT IS YOUR HEALTH GOAL?

So much dialog around health and nutrition strikes me as hot air and egotistical positioning; who is right, who is wrong, and who is smarter. I have absolutely no interest in any of it.

What I am interested in is this: to live until I am 96 years old, pharmaceutical free, pain free, disease free, and with all my organs intact.

That's it. That is my health goal, the reason I do all of this. My objective is not to live forever, or even a couple of centuries; 96 is good enough.

I mention my personal health goal because I have found that having one is helpful in navigating through the decisions any of us need to make when we discover the diet/disease, diet/symptom connection.

The number one reason anyone does a cleansing program is to lose some current symptom. And for now, that's a good enough goal. But once you lose your symptom, it will be helpful to come up with a bigger overall aim. Where do you want to go? What is the end desire?

BE PREPARED FOR THE UPSET

Because a large majority of people who heal themselves through diet will go through the same sequence of emotions that most everyone else goes through, I want to warn you beforehand: as your symptom starts to go away, be prepared to be pissed off. Losing your symptoms through a change of food will make you ask, why the hell weren't you told about this? Why the lies? All of these experts, all this money, all those expensive reports and tests and hospitals and seven-year university degrees, all this waste of resources and time, all the suffering, and not a single expert said to you: *"It's your food. Stop eating what you're eating, and start eating something different."*

I don't have any words of wisdom for how to deal with this upset. I am no therapist and this book isn't designed to help in that manner. Just know that your outrage and upset will play a very large role in helping spread the truth about basic human biology, and the true cost of being told that we're victims, not self-creators.

Every person that heals themselves through a change of diet will affect about 50 people around them. Your friends and family will see the difference. You will tell your coworkers about the process you went through to get healthy, to lose the Crohn's, the IBS, the Rosacea. And as some of those people start to apply these principles to their own health, they in turn will each affect 50 people around them. And on and on it goes. And that is the ultimate intent of this book: to bring common sense back to our understanding of how health works. One person at a time.

CHAPTER 4

What to eat during a cleanse & why

Internal cleansing is a protocol for healing that has been used in many cultures around the world, and throughout history. While there are variations, one of the common threads that link them all is their choice of foods: during a cleansing phase, all cultures chose a diet lower on the food chain; meaning, a plant-based diet. They saw that cleansing occurs best by lowering—or even completely removing— foods that come from animals, such as flesh foods and dairy.

Why is this? Part of the reason lies in looking at one of the main biological factors for why cleansing works. It is an internal process most commonly called autolyzation, a $10 word meaning "self-digestion." Autolyzation (or autolysis) is the "metabolizing of tissues and cells in an organism by actions produced within the organism itself." In other words, cleansing burns up the metabolic waste, toxins, mucus and gunk that are left behind in a body that has gotten clogged up. This left behind gunk is one of the main reasons for lowered functionality of our organs, like the liver, kidneys, and heart. When we hear of studies that tell us "a change in diet can reverse heart disease," they are talking about autolyzation: the body's ability to digest itself, once it's given a break from a diet rich in complex, sludge-producing foods.

ON ANIMAL FOODS

Animal foods—fish, meat, dairy—are very powerful building foods. They take more steps to digest and break down, and in a body already overloaded with metabolic waste, they can often times add to the pile. So, during your cleanse, you'll see that many of the recipes choose a more plant-based diet. This allows the body to burn through the mucus and sludge.

Contrary to what you may have heard, your body is completely capable of living (thriving, actually) on its own stored substances via this autolysis. We can stop worrying about "getting enough protein," at least during a cleansing period. We instead need a section of time in which we decompose and burn through the cells and tissues which are aged, damaged, diseased, weakened, dead, or downright toxic.

If you have never gone a month in your life without animal foods, I'm going to suggest you do a 100% plant-based cleanse. Not because it's right or wrong, but simply because it will probably give you better and faster results. It's also just a good experiment to try.

At the same time, some people don't do as well on a completely 100% plant-based diet as others. For instance, if you are a personal trainer, or a very physically active person who burns more calories than all the people in one office complex combined, you may find that you do better by adding some animal foods. That's fine. Bodies are fully capable of experiencing a massive jump in health and the overall effects of cleansing while still using some animal foods. History has proven this.

This is heresy to many cleansing practitioners, to even suggest animal foods during a cleansing phase. But over and over again, I see a certain type of person who actually get better results during their cleanse by adding a bit of animal foods to their broths and soups, an egg here and there. To not acknowledge this is to not be paying attention.

If you decide you are one of these people who will do better using a bit of animal foods during this cleansing program, there are some strong suggestions we recommend:

1. No dairy foods, period. It is too mucus forming. You will not experience cleansing if you eat dairy food. This includes milk, yogurt, kefir, cheese, and anything else that has come from an animal's udders. If you have never

weaned yourself and lived for a few months without some animal's breast milk, then you have no idea of its effects on your thinking and your emotions. It's time to give it a break.

2. No eating meat by itself. No steak or fish dinners. Instead, make your animal products 5-10 % of a total meal. Put some in a stir fry. Put pieces into a soup so that it makes up the broth. Think energetics. Not volume.

3. Choose only pure and organic. This is not a point open for discussion. If you doubt the dangers inherent in our current animal-food industry, you need to do some more reading. You need to locate uncontaminated organic, pure and clean sources of animal foods, even more so than with vegetables and fruits. Find sources that are clear of contamination, drugs, antibiotics, and cruelty. Don't use farm-raised fish, go for the wild variety (especially in salmon). Know where and how your animals were raised. What were they fed? What was their environment? How were they treated?

4. If you use animal foods during the cleanse, you must sweat often each week. Animal food is powerful medicine, much more than we acknowledge. It creates high energy, high heat, and no food on earth is more complex. If you are not naturally physically active, I suggest going very light on the animal foods, or doing a 100% plant-based cleanse.

5. Last, question your deeply ingrained beliefs about protein, and your need for it. This doesn't mean that your beliefs are wrong, and in fact may very well be right; each of our bodies is different, and this is not a book that is trying to turn us all into vegetarians. That's not the point. It's simply that a cleanse is a time to let the body come to a new conclusion. Don't limit the answers by eating a diet you've been eating for your entire life.

OTHER REQUIREMENTS

During a cleanse, besides preparing meals that are in the Recipe section, you want to make sure you are also doing the following:

DAILY REHYDRATION:

Learning to drink more water is a habit that you must learn during a cleanse. It is a critical step to flushing the cells. Use the following formula:

take your body weight, divide it in half, and drink that amount of water in ounces. For example, if you weigh 100 pounds, drink at least 50 ounces of pure water each day; if you weigh 200 pounds, drink at least 100 ounces of pure water each day.

DAILY REMINERALIZE:

Every day, be use foods that are very high in trace minerals. There are many sources, and two of the easiest and best are Celtic gray sea salt and algae, both salt and fresh water varieties. You can also get encapsulated wild bluegreen algae, chlorella, and spirulina at your local health food stores.

DAILY REBACTERIALIZE

One of the most injurious sins of our current cultural diet is that it is devoid of cultured, fermented foods. You may think, "hey, I eat pickles." Perhaps, but I'd bet money that they are pasteurized, which kills the friendly bacteria found in them. So, from here on out, you want to eat some cultured, fermented foods every day, in order to bring healthy bacteria into your digestive tract. Use encapsulated bacteria (also called probiotics) as well. See the section on Fermented Foods for ideas.

DAILY REENZYMIZE

Enzymes are the tiny microscopic part of foods that act as catalysts to help break down and digest. However, when we heat foods past about 115 degrees, there are no more enzymes. This doesn't mean cooked foods are bad, but an enzyme-rich diet can speed up the internal cleansing process. Each day, eat uncooked foods that are rich in enzymes. Like friendly bacteria, enzymes can be found in capsules, and used as a supplement to your diet.

PHYSICAL TRANSFORMERS

In the original 28-Day Regeneration Program, I used an entire audio CD to describe some powerful actions—called *Physical Transformers*—outside of diet that also aid in cleansing the cells. During a cleanse, try to do at least one of them every day. They are:

Skin Brushing— vigorously brush your skin before or during a shower or bath. Your skin is your largest elimination organ, and it needs all the breathing it can get.

Rehydrating— During your cleanse, drink 3 to 4 quarts of pure spring water a day. One of the important reasons for rehydrating is lymph, the body's internal garbage transportation system. The lymph system is the often overlooked set of vessels used to transport metabolic waste out of the body. During a cleanse, the lymph system can become overwhelmed with old, necrotic material. Extra water is a key to helping it move along. Buy a bottle, somewhere around the size of a gallon. This will be your official rehydration jug. Fill it each day, and drink it empty each day. It is really the only way you are going to be able to measurably know how much water you are using. If you don't have access to spring water, then filter your tap water with a carbon filter.

Sauna Rounds— Most people have been in a sauna before, but few have used them in a guided, cell rejuvenating way. Saunas require some conditioning, in order to get past that "I'm hot and uncomfortable" feeling. This suffering comes about because the skin is not conditioned… it's not opening and closing to allow the sweat to flow. The key is to do what I call "sauna rounds."

Start with a light skin brushing—this will help to get things going. Now go into the sauna for about 5-10 minutes. Once you're sweating a bit, step out and take a cold "plunge" for a count of 10 or 20 (either under a shower or a bath filled with cold water). It's only a few seconds, but that contraction of the skin, that squeezing of the lymph system, is very important.

That's round one. Now hop back into the sauna. This time, you'll start to notice that you break a sweat faster, and you're going to sweat more. After 5 or 10 minutes, jump out into another 10-20 second cold plunge. Skin brush if you want, then start Round 3. Work up to 2 or 3 of these "rounds." If you need to rest between sessions, just lie down outside the sauna for a while. Stay hydrated. Always have plenty of water.

Most people think that owning their own sauna for detoxifying and regenerating is a luxury they can't afford. Not true. Like a juicer and other health-giving tools, portable and lightweight Far Infrared saunas are now available for under $2000. I use one regularly. Whether you live in an apartment, or mobile home, or large house, Far Infrared saunas are now designed to be stored in any apartment closet. Check our site, www. HowHealthWorks.com for options. Members get a deep discount that more than pays for an entire year of membership cost.

Alkalinizing Baths— Toss a cup of sea salt (cheap is okay) or cup of baking soda into a bath. Get in and slowly increase the heat until you are sweating. The object is to make the outside water more alkaline than the body and blood itself. It is easy, relaxing, and very powerful when combined with skin brushing.

Cleansing Bodywork— There are a few types of physical and energetic manipulations that can aid in cleansing. The best I've found are deep tissue, Thai and Shiatsu massage, Rolfing, visceral manipulation, and acupuncture. Try to get a few sessions in during your cleansing period.

Colon hydrotherapy— Colon hydrotherapy involves the gentle introduction of a few gallons of purified water—sometimes infused with minerals or chlorophyll—into the colon using a small tube that is placed a few inches into the rectum. This internal water therapy has a history that goes back at least a few hundred years. Hippocrates mentions a type of enema in his writing. Lewis and Clark's physician, before their long voyage across America in 1803, gave the men instructions on the use of internal water therapy for reversing the onset of fever and illness. As late as the 1930s, hospitals used colon irrigation machines as part of their standard practice. Colon hydrotherapy can be done in two ways: by going to a professional colon hydrotherapist, or self-administered, using a device called a colema board. For further information, see the e-book *Advanced Colon Cleansing* at the www.HowHealthWorks.com site.

Cardiovascular Workout— There are two reasons you want to work out during a cleansing period. The first is the cleansing effect of sweating and moving our blood by elevating the heart rate. The second and often overlooked effect is the health-producing changes that occur in our hormones and chemistry. Working out increases our sense of wellbeing and promotes a higher self-esteem. Three times a week, do some form of physical exercise.

These seven Physical Transformers are ancient and have been used for centuries. They help cleanse and purge the body, both internally and externally, by keeping the natural pathways of metabolism open. I have personally shortened flu and cold symptoms with these tools. They help move the body's lymph, improve skin, and revitalize energy and mental clarity.

CHAPTER 5

The Tools

M ost kitchens are not designed to produce health. Instead, they look like an advertisement for fast foods, filled with empty calories that clog the body and weaken our immunity. So one of the first important steps to a successful health turnaround will be preparing your kitchen as though it were the *real* center of your health care program. Because it is.

As you deepen your understanding of the diet/disease, diet/symptom connection, you will start to recognize that the source of healing is not your country's national health plan, but your kitchen. As such, you need to prepare the space to work for, not against you. You want to make it easy to prepare the nutrition that will regenerate your body back to health. This requires some tools and a pantry.

Don't be overwhelmed by the following list. You can do a cleansing program without a completely decked-out kitchen—you can even do it on the back of a 1962 Ford Econoline van with just a handful of foods, one pan, and a sharp Swiss Army knife while traveling across America (as Scott did in the mid 1970s). If you are on a tight budget, you can get by with the basics. If you are going to cleanse mainly through the health food store or deli method, much of the following won't necessarily apply. But to give you an idea, read through the following sections.

In carpentry, there's a saying: you are only as good as your tools. Well, the same can be said for a kitchen. The tools you see below are all the kind that, within a minute of first using them, you will experience a moment of awe, as in, "Wow. *This* makes food preparation fun!" And that's exactly the feeling you want to have when you step into your healing kitchen.

There is no need to purchase all of these tools right away. Just know that most of them will last a lifetime, so add them as you can. Start with a good Japanese cutting knife, then get a pot or two, then a juicer, and so on.

I have a passion for scouring the world and finding not only the best source for each of these tools, but the best price. So before you buy, check out our tools web page where we post the most current place to buy the best cleansing tools at the best prices. We update it regularly. It's located at:

www.howhealthworks.com/tools/

CREATING A
SYMPTOM-REPAIRING KITCHEN

JAPANESE VEGETABLE KNIFE

All food preparation starts with the knife, and in the world of cutting vegetables, there is no equal when it comes to Japanese vegetable knives. Second place isn't even close. The reasons for this become apparent the very first time you pick one up and start slicing. It's in 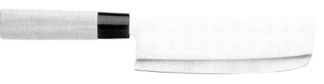 their balance, the thin blade, and the way the blade cuts. For those who have always used meat knives, the contrast is an immediate pleasure.

Like most fine tools, the price varies greatly. Fortunately, it is possible to find inexpensive Japanese knives that will work perfectly for years, in the range of

$30 (and it's easy to spend $90 and more). I still have the first carbon steel knife with a bamboo handle that I bought for $29 in 1984, and it still holds an edge.

A couple of things to look for: choose a metal that will rust. While you can get stainless steel Japanese vegetable knives (I own two of them), they are difficult to sharpen, so go with the softer carbon steel metal. Also, for your first knife, look for a profile like the one pictured here. Note that it has a very slight curve along the sharpened edge. While you can find ones with a perfectly flat edge, I find cutting easier if there is a slight bow along the cutting edge.

JUICER

One of the basic requirements of this program is to drink fresh vegetable juice every day. Unless you live near a juice bar, you will need to beg, borrow, or purchase a home juicer. Modern juicers also double as tools for making fresh nut butters and the delicious and raw and quick gazpacho-style soup recipes.

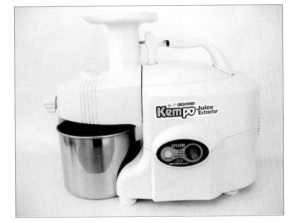

If you're new to juicing, borrow one from a friend. Once you feel the benefits, buy your own. There are three distinct and valid ways to do that:

1. Buy a used one on eBay. Use the two ideas below to guide you.

2. Buy a starter juicer. These will run from $50-150, and will last a year or two before burning out. This can be a quite suitable way to test out juicing in your own body.

3. Buy a juicer that will outlive you. These will start around $200 (for the Champion) and can go up to the $390-$600 range (for the twin-helical gear models). There are juicers priced beyond this, but for home juicing, they are unnecessary.

Having experimented with a dozen models over the years, I think the finest juicers on the market right now are the twin-helical gear units. There are about six models to choose from, available in both 110 and 220v, and competitively priced throughout the Internet. Regardless of the hype you will read, they are all good, and all made by two extremely reputable manufacturers in Korea, and will all last for ten years or more. Further,

1. Their extremely slow turning speeds (less than 180 RPM) lead to less oxidation, so juice is fresher and lasts longer.

2. The twin gear models are the only ones on the market that juice wheatgrass without the fibers clogging the system. This means that people no longer need to own two separate juicers.

3. Easy cleanup, and takes less than 3 minutes.

That said, use whatever juicer you can get. They all basically work and get the job done.

HEALTHY COOKWARE

It's time to throw out all aluminum and non-stick kitchenware, and get pots and pans made from materials that can't make your sick. The main substances to look for are, in no particular order:

1. **Stainless steel**
2. **Cast Iron**
3. **Glass**

STAINLESS STEEL

There are many companies now making high quality stainless steel pots and pans, and with the Internet, you can often find great deals.

By itself, stainless steel does not spread heat very well. This is why you will find that stainless cookware manufacturers bond the bottom surface with another material, usually aluminum or copper. While these two metals should not come in contact with food, they are superb heat displacers, and are perfect when sandwhiched between layers of stainless steel.

For starters, get a four-quart sauce pan, and a ten inch frying pan, both with lids. Get professional weight, which is usually measured as 18/10 stainless.

Cast Iron

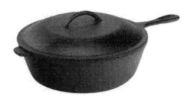

These are inexpensive, readily available, heats food evenly and lasts a lifetime. The two most useful items are a ten-inch skillet for sauteing and a deep pan for making soups.

Another great version of cast iron is the enameled versions. Much more expensive, but equally useful and safe.

Pyrex Glassware Pans

One of the hidden tools of a healing kitchen is actually one that isn't being manufactured anymore, at least in the United States. It is the Pyrex line of glass pots and pans. These are a pleasure to cook with, and are completely non-toxic.

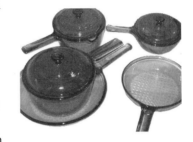

Because millions of units were made in the mid-twentieth century, they are still available on the used market, often in mint condition, and often very cheap. The best place to search for these great kitchen pieces is eBay. Entire seven-piece sets can often be had for $25, plus shipping. We have purchased some really nice sets, and there are often hundreds of auctions going on. And shhh... don't tell anyone how great these are for the natural cook. We don't want the prices to start going up...

GRAIN COOKER

Whole grains are a part of every long-living culture. Learning to cook them is a simple skill required of anyone wanting a long, healthy life. While a pressure cooker (see next tool) gives us more control, an automatic grain cooker makes prepping and eating grains easy. It is the way to go for those with no time to spend in the kitchen, or bachelors, students or kids who want to learn something easy to eat. How easy is a grain cooker? Two steps:

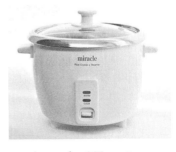

1. Place water, grain, and a pinch of salt in the stainless steel inner pot.

2. Push the ON button.

That's it. Automatic grain cookers turn themselves off at the right time, and then switch to warm mode. You can cook rice, barley, quinoa, oats and most other whole grains without thinking about it.

NOTE: be very careful about which grain cooker you purchase. The vast majority of them use an inner cooking pot made from aluminum or some kind of non-stick chemical surface. Some units fool you by having a stainless steel exterior, but the material contacting your food is Teflon or aluminum. If you can't find a healthy grain cooker, check at our cleansing tools page, http://www.howhealthworks.com/tools/.

GARLIC PEELER

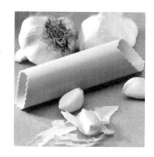

Out of all the tools, this has one of the higher "wow" factors. A six-dollar tube of silicone rubber that strips the peel from garlic cloves by rolling it on the counter. You have to see it to believe it.

FLAME TAMER

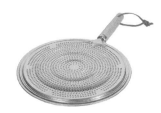

A four dollar device that sits between your flame and your pot. Spreads and softens the heat, making it easy to keep heat on a dish for hours, such as with overnight oats, and beans that you want to cook for 4 or 5 hours. An invaluable, simple tool.

HAND FOOD CHOPPER

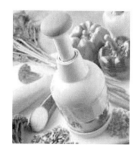

For chopping a cup or two of vegetables in a hurry, this tool has become one of my favorites. I first saw it in action at a friend's home a few years ago, and became immediately intrigued. Just grab any vegetable small enough to fit under the cylinder, and rapidly depress the plunger a few times. The durable rotating blades chop through vegetables and nuts, but are especially handy with aromatic onions and garlic.

I'm always trying out different brands of tools, and these food choppers are no exception. In this category, only one has proven to be worth getting: Pampered Chef's Food Chopper. It is priced at about $30. Like the blender wand, you will use it every day.

PRESSURE COOKER

If you want the best tasting beans and grains, then you will want to get a modern pressure cooker.

In the early years, pressure cookers were the things that occasionally blew up in mom's kitchen. Fortunately, modern units have made them

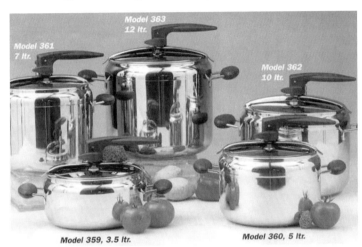

Model 363 12 ltr.
Model 361 7 ltr.
Model 362 10 ltr.
Model 359, 3.5 ltr.
Model 360, 5 ltr.

not only safe to use, but shorten cooking times and increase the flavor of our basic whole foods. Instead of simmering garbanzo beans for 8 hours, you can pressure cooker them for 90 minutes.

Your first pressure cooker can be the last you will ever buy. I bought my first Aeternum (pictured above) pressure cooker in 1984, and it's still going strong over 20 years later. And the thick stainless steel still shines like a mirror.

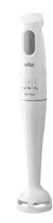

BLENDER WAND

This is a must-have item. And at around $30, it's a screaming value. Purée soups in a flash, make whole-grain cream cereal, create dressings that will wow anyone. And most importantly, it is tiny and cleans up in seconds: just unscrew the base, rinse under hot water, and rack dry. We use ours nearly every day.

There are many manufacturers to choose from, we have tried them all. They are about equal in durability and cost, so just buy the one currently on sale. Since purchasing our first one in the early 1990s, our heavy, massive, expensive and chore-to-clean Cuisinart food processor has largely gathered dust.

FOOD PROCESSOR

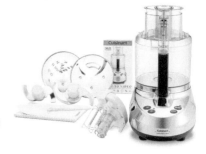

Now that I've trashed large, heavy, pain-to-clean, dust-collecting food processors, Joann is forcing me to put in a good word about them. She says, *"Food processors have very strong motors, which are perfect for pureeing foods, allowing you to create a smooth texture from beans, fruits, vegetables, seeds, nuts and herbs. They are the best tool to make pestos, spreads, dips or foods where you usually need to first blend the bulky food, then add the liquid. This allows you to adjust the liquid as needed. They are different than a blender wand or stick, which you will typically use for more liquid-based foods such as soups, drinks and sauces."*

SLOW COOKER (CROCK POT)

One of the meals that is often left out of a fast food society is the deeply nourishing stew. It can be a main source of energy and fuel, especially during a cleanse. While stews and soups can be made in a large pot over the stove, a crock pot makes it easier. Due to the nature of a slow cooker, there is no need to stir the food. In fact, taking the lid off is frowned upon by crock pot purists. This combination of no stirring, no lid lifting, low heat, and long hours of cooking can make the most delicious meals during a largely vegetarian cleansing experience.

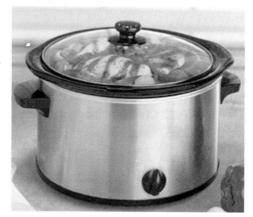

HARSCH FERMENTING POT

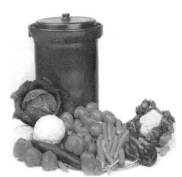

Every once in a while, someone in some country at some point comes up with the perfect food, or the perfect tool, that becomes a timeless, must-have item. The Harsch fermenting pot is one of those perfect tools that everyone who grasps the diet/disease, diet/symptom connection should own.

There is no easier way to create your own fermented vegetables than with these German-designed ceramic "harsch" fermenting pots. The secret behind them is their clever water sealing top that allows fermentation gasses to escape without allowing air to enter the crock pot. Fermenting vegetables can be a bit tricky, but with this specially designed pot, it is impossible to go wrong, and you will make perfect fermented vegetables the very first time.

How Health Works imports these beautiful hand-crafted stoneware fermenting pots directly from a potter's factory in Germany where they've been manufactured for over 70 years. Each pot is fired at 1200 degrees and finished with a lead-free glaze suitable for all vegetable fermenting. Some advantages:

- NO SMELL—You can make fermented vegetables (kimchi, sauerkraut, etc) right in your kitchen and have absolutely no smells during the fermenting process.
- FAST—7 to 12 days, and you have the world's best cultured foods.
- CHEAP HEALTH— salt and veggies, perhaps a couple of spices. That's it.
- NO MOLD— Sealed water top speeds up the fermenting process and prevents mold (very common with other methods)
- BRILLIANT DESIGN— Its design allows air to escape but none to enter.
- WEIGHTS INCLUDED— Includes two lead-free ceramic weights which fit perfectly inside the crock pot to always keep the vegetables under the brine.
- EASY TO CLEAN— critical for good fermenting. Just wipe down with hot water. Extremely wide mouth for easy access.

If you do not have a Harsch pot, just use a large glass container.

SALAD SPINNER

Salad dressing will cling to dry salad (or cooked leafy greens) instead of sinking to the bottom of the bowl. Salad spinners work by spinning all of the water off your produce. You can splurge for the good ones (around $30), but we have found the cheap ones work fine as well. Joann has used a five-dollar model for over four years, and is plenty happy with it. Her spinner trick: wash greens, spin, and store them in bags in the refrigerator. Then they are is ready in a moment's notice.

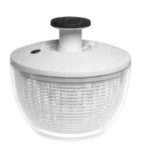

SURIBACHI

A suribachi is a Japanese mortar used along with a wooden pestle to grind seeds and herbs, and to mix ingredients into pastes. As you can see by the close-up lower photo, the inside surface is rough, which helps grind and combine foods. We have two of them; one is used solely for grinding Celtic sea salt. It is actually a very fun tool to use, and whenever we have guests for dinner, I always try to leave something to grind or combine. It gives them something to do while we're talking and doing the final meal preparation.

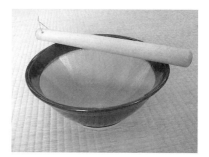

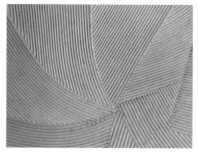

CHAPTER 6

The Pantry

pan·try *(pan'tree) A small room or closet, usually off a kitchen, where canned, bottled, dried, and other food items are stored.*

Most kitchens we see are designed to make it hard to prepare food. Olive oil is purchased in 6 ounce bottles, grains in two cup bags, and when the recipe calls for one onion, the person buys... one onion. For those eating for health, this is crazy making. You can not nourish yourself in this manner. You need to make a pantry.

A well-stocked pantry lends itself to the inspiration of a good cook. Adapting recipes to your taste buds as well as to whatever is in your cupboards is half the fun of cooking, and half the source of creativity.

As with the Tools section, do not let this list overwhelm you. Don't panic and think you have to get all these items right now. This is a list you can slowly build and use as a reference, even years from now. If you can only put together the bare minimum, with access to good clean water, good Celtic sea salt, olive oil, and some produce, beans and grains, you can do this cleanse. In other words, not having a pantry is no excuse for not cleansing.

On the next page is a comprehensive list for a fully stocked pantry. The best way to organize yourself it to think in terms of categories. All categories are listed together, and then the details are in the following section.

Pantry Categories

- ❖ Grains
- ❖ Beans
- ❖ Vegetables
- ❖ Oils & Fats
- ❖ Nuts & Seeds
- ❖ Fermented Foods
- ❖ Sea Vegetables
- ❖ Beverages
- ❖ Condiments & Seasonings
- ❖ Herbs & Spices
- ❖ Fruits & Dried Fruits
- ❖ Sweeteners
- ❖ Freezer & Packaged & Canned Foods
- ❖ Superfoods & the Three Rs
- ❖ Crunch & Road Food
- ❖ Foods to Avoid

❖ GRAINS

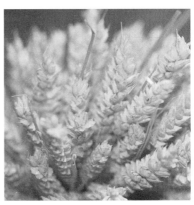

Whole grains are often associated with anything related to carbohydrates, refined or otherwise. Because of this, it is important that we examine **Carbo-phobia,** the most recent and bizarre approach to health currently in America. If you are caught up in carbo-phobia, please be sure to read about it in the next section.

When we talk about grains in relationship to healing and cleansing, we are always talking about whole grains—meaning, the entire seed. The most common whole grains are:

• Amaranth	• Oatmeal groats (not rolled)
• Barley	• Quinoa (keen'•wah)
• Buckwheat groats	• Brown Rice (any whole variety)
• Jobs tears (a type of barley)	• Teff
• Kamut	• Wheat Berries
• Millet	

There are also two grain products that fit into a cleansing lifestyle:

• Essene or Manna bread (sprouted, enzymatically active)	• Mochi (mashed and pounded brown rice cake)

Whole grains are the body's best source of fuel. Nothing tops them; absolutely nothing. All long-living cultures (back as far as the Sumerians, 2500 BC) figured that out and used grains as a staple of their diets. Pound per pound, whole grains also happened to be the most economical way to feed yourself and your family.

However, what most people associate with the word "grain" is not whole grains at all, but bread, crackers, whole-wheat muffins, bran, noodles, pasta shaped so that it looks like rice, grits, bulgar, flattened or cut oats, or couscous. None of these are whole grains, and during a cleansing program, you want to avoid them. While these partial grain products can be fun and tasty, they are often the cause of many sludge-producing problems and symptoms. Along with bad oils and dairy foods, nothing gums up the inner works like fractionated grains or flour products. You will see this yourself within the first few weeks of eliminating them entirely from your diet.

Pantry: Grains are best stored in airtight glass containers. They also look beautiful that way, and allow you to store and stack them anywhere in your kitchen or pantry. Get at least a few pounds at a time.

Essene bread deserves special attention. This is because it is not really bread as we know it, and it is about the only one that works during a cleanse. Instead of ground flour, it is made from fresh sprouted whole grains, simply squashed together and then baked at a low enough temperature that the enzymes remain active. The temperature is so low that freezing it is the only way for the bakers to get it to your local health food store without it spoiling. So, Joann and I suggest stocking up on this bread in your freezer (you can get it in cases of 12). The best company we've found is Nature's Path (www.NaturesPath.com).

Mochi is a condensed cake made from pounded rice. It comes in half-inch thick packages about six inches square. Like Essene bread, it survives nicely in the freezer, making it a great last-minute method to get whole grains into your meal. Be sure to only choose the whole grain varieties. It can be fried or baked.

❖ BEANS

After decades of going to potluck dinners and dealing with the after effects of undercooked bean dishes, I am convinced that hardly anyone in our culture was ever taught how to prepare beans so that they are digestible. Not presoaked, not cooked nearly long enough, and not combined with the right foods, it's no wonder people avoid them.

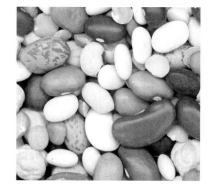

This is a nutritional error. Beans (also known as legumes) are an ancient stable energy source, and help prevent blood-sugar swings. They are one of the better sources of plant-based minerals, notably iron. They are also high-quality protein, and are showing to be good dietary support for those with digestive-tract problems. In worldwide studies that examined the correlations between food intake and heart disease, researchers have found that higher legume consumption was associated with up to an 80% reduction in heart attacks. According to Oriental medicine, beans tonify and strengthen the kidneys and support the reproductive system.

HOW TO MAKE BEANS DIGESTIBLE

So if we are going to talk about beans, we need to learn first how to prepare them. Below are the tricks that work. Start by following these steps:

1. Soak beans overnight. No other single tip will make as much difference! Presoaking has been found to reduce the amount of sugars known as *raffinose*, which can cause flatulence. Presoaking can be done in two ways. In both methods, start by adding about three cups of water per one cup of beans. Then boil the beans for 10 minutes, and let sit for four hours. Or, soak the beans overnight.

2. Discard the soaking water and rinse the beans.

3. Add the soaked, rinsed beans to water. Use approximately 3 cups of water to each cup of beans. Bring to boil. During the first 15 minutes of simmering, skim off any foam that accumulates at the top.

4. Now add a piece of kombu seaweed (a thick form of kelp). Kombu is called "nature's MSG" because it contains the amino acid called glutamate, a tenderizer that helps digest beans, and also adds flavor. You can also add bay leaf, onion or carrot while you are cooking to impart flavor.

5. Do not simmer any bean for less than two hours. Four to six hours is better. Overnight simmering is good, too. I have yet to eat an overcooked bean.

6. Alternatively, pressure cook your beans. Do not fill more than half full. Add a teaspoon of oil to prevent foam. Seal up the pressure cooker and bring up to pressure. Once pressure has been reached, cook the beans for 90 to 120 minutes. After the time is up, let the pressure come down naturally. Open your cooker and drain your beans.

7. Cheat: buy canned beans. Organic canned or glass-jarred beans are one of the few places where precooked produce actually works to your advantage. But there is one strong caveat: purchase only products that contain essentially water, salt, and the whole bean. I would avoid those that have added soy, safflower or canola oil, textured soy, autolyzed yeast, sweeteners and flours (yes, even if they are organic). There are now some very diligent bean canning companies, such as Eden™, Westbrae™, and Amy's™.

Other tips for making beans a flatulence-free experience:

Watch your food combining. Don't add sweeteners or fruit to beans or bean dishes.

Certain spices counteract the production of intestinal gas. Fortunately, they all taste great in bean dishes. Try fenugreek seeds, marjoram, ginger root, cumin, caraway seeds, turmeric, parsley and black pepper.

Cook beans thoroughly before adding acidic foods, like tomatoes, lemon, and vinegar. Don't add salt until the last few minutes.

Eat small portions of beans to build up your body's ability to process them. Your body will develop the enzymes to break down beans.

While combining beans with grains is popular in many countries, I find that the combination makes the meal harder to digest. Try separating beans from grains if you're having problems with digestion.

As mentioned above: if you pressure cook your beans, add a tablespoon of olive oil to prevent the vent from becoming clogged.

Anything that increases the body's enzymes or friendly bacteria will increase your ability to digest beans, and any other meal. Pay attention to rebuilding your internal friendly flora, as outlined in the first section.

Any bean is a good bean. Here is a starter list

Black/White Beans	Anasazi Beans
• Black-eye peas	• Adzuki Beans (aka Aduki)
• Garbanzo Beans (aka Chickpea)	• Kidney Beans
• Lentils Beans	• Navy Beans
• Pinto Beans	• Fava
• Cannellini Beans	• Split peas

Lentils, chickpeas (garbanzos), and adzuki beans are often easier to digest than other beans. But we all digest differently, so the key will be to find the beans that you digest particularly well.

Pantry: Like grains, beans are best stored in airtight glass containers, and add beauty to your kitchen. Get as many varieties as you can to store and display.

And finally, from one of the best books on legumes, *Romancing the Bean,* by author Joann Saltzman:

"Always soak beans before cooking. An inch of kombu sea vegetable per cup of dry bean helps break down the secondary compounds that inhibit digestion. Don't add salt until the very end. But the most important part of cooking a bean is to make sure it is velvety soft. A digestible bean is soft like butter inside a thin skin which defines its shape. A crunchy bean will fight the body, producing intestinal pain or gas.

"Last, don't be seduced by their wonderful taste: stick with a reasonable serving of a quarter to a half cup of cooked beans with your meal."

❖ VEGETABLES

Stocking vegetables for a cleansing lifestyle is easy: with the exception of nightshades, use them all. Experiment. Use what is in season. Most people's biggest challenge will be to expand their repertoire beyond the five or six they grew up with. Below is a short list, but there are many more:

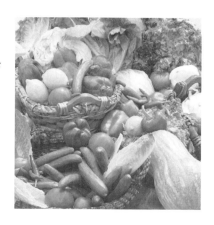

ALWAYS KEEP IN STOCK:

• Onions	• Garlic
• Leafy greens	• Carrots
• Ginger root	• Cabbage

OTHER VEGETABLES

• Cabbages: Napa, Bok Choy, red and green cabbage	• Mushrooms: portobello, cremini, button, shiitake
• Squashes, especially dark yellow	• Cucumber
• Celery	• Avocado
• Broccoli	• Okra
• Kohlrabi	• Spring onion (aka green onion)
• Sweet corn	

ROOTS & TUBERS

• Carrots	• Onions
• Garlic	• Daikon radish
• Red radish	• Beets
• Parsnips	• Turnips
• Sweet potatoes	• Yams
• Taro root	• Burdock
• Ginger root	

Leafy Greens

• Lettuce & leafy salad greens	• Kale, collards, mustard greens,
• Parsley	• Arugula
• Endive	• Fennel
• Watercress	• Dandelion greens

Nightshades

While most any vegetable is a good vegetable, there is a certain category of them worth some caution. These are the ones belonging to the nightshade family.

Nightshades are some of the most popular vegetables in the world, eaten every day by some people. Yet few are aware of the adverse symptoms that nightshades can have on our health, and therefore never associate those symptoms to their daily meal choices.

Nightshade is the common name given to a certain group of plants that belong to the *Solanum* genus. Nightshades have long been used as stimulants, narcotics, and pain relievers. Most Solanum plants are downright poisonous, such as belladonna, tobacco, datura, and mandrake.

However, there are a few that are used as food. The most common four are **potatoes**, **tomatoes**, **eggplant**, and **all peppers** (except black pepper).

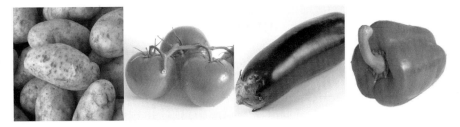

All nightshades contain strong alkaloids that have been associated with joint pain (osteoarthritis, rheumatoid arthritis, gout) skin problems (psoriasis, eczema), migraines, and nerve and muscle problems (twitching, trembling, shortness of breath). Some report sleep disturbance and wild dreams.

56

Dr. Norman Childers, Ph.D., from the Arthritis Nightshades Research Foundation says, *"Plants in the drug family, Solanaceae (nightshades) are an important causative factor in arthritis in sensitive people."*

In *Healing Psoriasis*, probably the best known cleansing book on psoriasis and eczema, author Dr. John Pagano shows case after case of people clearing their inflammatory symptoms through diet that excludes tomatoes, eggplant, potatoes and peppers.

Dr. Sherry Rogers, M.D., author of *Wellness Against All Odds*, says, *"For many, no relief comes until the diet has been totally free of all of these [nightshades] for at least 6-12 weeks. So you can appreciate why, if someone gives them up for a couple of weeks and sees no improvement, that he could easily be convinced to abandon the diet and indulge in his favorites again, never to discover the culprit."*

All of this has to be weighed with the knowledge that some cultures have used these four nightshades for centuries. And nightshade alkaloids can be reduced by 40 or 50 percent through cooking. Still, it is worth noting that for many people suffering from related symptoms, at least one of these four nightshades is eaten on a regular basis (and often grows in their garden). If you have any of the symptoms associated with nightshade consumption, notably physical pain or skin problems of any type, these vegetables would be the first foods that I would eliminate from my diet.

If you are suffering from joint pain or skin problems, I would eliminate all nightshades from your diet. In the case where they are one of the ingredients in the recipes here, simply leave them out, preparing the dish without them.

OXALIC ACID VEGETABLES

Oxalic acid is a mild toxin found in many plants, and when in the wrong balance, it can cause health problems. It can irritate the stomach and intestines. It binds with iron as well as calcium and either leeches it from the body or forms oxalate crystals that remain and further irritate the digestive tract.

Not all vegetables high in oxalic acid have these effects. In some high oxalic acid plants, there seems to be enough calcium, magnesium and other buffering compounds in the vegetable that balance out this acid's effect. For instance, chives have 1.50 grams per 100 grams; parsley is even higher, at 1.7 grams per 100 grams. Those are relatively high numbers, but no one has ever reported an oxalic acid reaction with those plants. In fact, those plants are often associated with helping to alkalinize a meal. They are both welcome in a cleansing diet.

Yet there are definitely some plants that should be watched, especially for those suffering from any bone loss or body and joint pain. These are:

- Rhubarb (NEVER eat rhubarb leaves)
- Beet leaves (.6 grams per 100 grams)
- Swiss chard
- Spinach (.9 grams per 100 grams)
- Sorrel

A couple of interesting notes about oxalic acid: the gritty feeling you get if you eat rhubarb pie (high in oxalic acid) and milk (high in calcium) is the precipitation, right there in your mouth, of the acid and calcium. Also, oxalic acid reduces iron compounds, and is therefore used in metal polishes, furniture stain removers, and even pen ink.

THE ENERGETICS OF FOOD

With the above lists of nightshades and oxalic acid vegetables, it is important not to write these off as "Bad plants. Bad!" As as we noted with parsley and chives, you can not isolate one ingredient out of hundreds in order to determine how that vegetable affects your body. There are too many other factors that come in to play when determining how to live to 96 years old, drug and pain and symptom free. **What these lists do is allow us to pay attention.** They are markers made by others who have noted the energetics of those plants. Our job is to pay attention and see what works in our own body, and in our own healing process.

❖ OILS & FATS

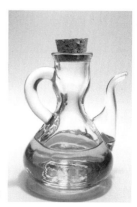

Unless you have been living under a rock for the past decade, you will have noticed that fats and oils (also known as lipids) have gotten plenty of press, probably more than any single nutrient in the current concerns of diet and human health.

And for good reason. Blocked arteries and malfunctions of the heart—together known as heart disease—are now the single largest killer in America. No one doubts that fats play a roll in this. The question is: what kinds of fat? In what form? Which fats heal us, and which fats are killing us?

THE OIL MUCK

There is currently no single greater confusing subject in all of nutrition than fats and oils. One of the reasons for this is the ever-growing language around fat. Look at this partial list of words now associated with the fat research: saturated and un-saturated; monounsaturated, mono-glycerides hydrogenat-ed, polyunsaturated, cis-fatty and trans-fatty. You also have your monoglycerides, di-glyceride, and let's not forget tri-glycerides. To this mess, start adding the really self-explanatory terms of LDL, HDL, HDL-1, HDL-2, and why not, HDL-3.

> *"There is no bigger health scandal. Cholesterol can strike terror in the hearts of misinformed people. The cholesterol scare is big business for doctors, laboratories, and drug companies. It is also a powerful marketing gimmick for manufacturers who can say their products are cholesterol-free."*
>
> UDO ERASMUS
> FATS THAT HEAL, FATS THAT KILL

THE CHOLESTEROL MUCK

To further the confusion, most of us have become familiar with the term cholesterol, which has been considered *the* marker for fat health in both our body and the foods we ingest. Cholesterol is a waxy substance manufactured by your body. It is a life-enhancing necessity, producing hormones such as estrogen and testosterone, and a key to rebuilding damaged cell membranes and brain and nerve tissue.

For decades, it has been suggested that everyone get their cholesterol levels checked regularly, based on the idea that the amounts we have in us can determine if we are healthy or not.

That is not so clear any more. People with high levels of cholesterol live to be old. People with low levels can die of heart disease. Our body seems to produce more cholesterol when we eat low-cholesterol food; conversely, our body seems to produce less when we eat too much high-cholesterol food.

USE HISTORY AND YOUR BRAIN

This confusion around fat and cholesterol is solid proof that when it comes to learning how to stay healthy, you will need to use your brain, common sense, and a bit of history, more than someone's facts and figures. What this means is that you and I are going to have to experiment a bit.

Fortunately, there are some guidelines that can help us choose what fats we put into our pantry:

Fats are good, and we need them.
If you value clear thinking, a nervous system that runs well, beautiful skin, emotions that make sense, avoiding obesity, a liver that remains clear of congestion, and the vitamins A, D, E, and K, then you need some fat every day.

> "It is simply wrong to blame fats for degenerative conditions. The scientific research and the historical data of tribal eating habits simply don't support the saturated fat and atherosclerosis theory of heart disease."
>
> DR. WILLIAM CAMPBELL DOUGLASS, M.D.

Fake fats are not good, and we need to avoid them like the plague.
I don't think there is another substance that wrecks health more than hydrogenated fat, which is any oil that has been processed through a chemical-hardening method to achieve stiffness or plasticity at room temperature. Hydrogenated and partially hydrogenated oils are found in nearly all packaged baked goods, chips, cakes, candies, microwave popcorn, any deep fried foods, and most any snack found in a box. Worse are the toxic "fat replacers" such as Olestra or Salatrim.

Let history be your guide
If epidemiological studies show that a certain population lives long healthy
lives, and uses certain oils, chances are good those oils are health-producing.

Get most of your fats from foods, nuts and seeds
Most liquid oils turn rancid once exposed to light, oxygen and heat, yet are
fine when consumed in their original whole form. Soybeans have a natural oil
in them that is high in lecithin and anti-cancer factors, yet it is nearly impossible to get liquid soybean oil that is stable and not rancid. This is the same
with most nut oils. Pumpkin seeds are a powerful anti-parasite, anti-fungal
additions to a cleansing diet, but I would not suggest getting it in liquid form.
Flax seeds are rich in essential fatty acids, yet its oil is highly unstable once it
is in a bottled form.

Just because it's vegetarian, doesn't mean it's good.
This will come as a surprise to many, but just because someone figures out
how to get oil out of a fairly non-oily plant, doesn't mean it's healthy. If a
plant or vegetable doesn't naturally feel oily in your hand, chances are good
that it took too much processing to squeeze out what's there. **I would avoid
the following popular vegetable oils:**

- Safflower oil
- Corn oil
- Canola oil
- Soybean oil
- Cottonseed oil
- Margarine (of any variety)

Just because it's saturated, doesn't mean it is bad for you.
Another recent surprise is finding out that not all saturated fats are bad for
us. The simple definition of saturated fat used to be "fats that are solid at
room temperature." It's now known that while raw coconut oil and artificially
hydrogenated Crisco-style vegetable fat are both solid at room temperatures,
they are quite different in their effect on human health. Clean-quality saturated fat has been found to be the preferred fuel for your heart, has powerful
antiviral, anti-cavity, and anti-fungal properties, and can actually help remove
plaque and artery buildup.

SUGGESTED OILS FOR EATING AND COOKING

Here are the main historically proven oils recommended for your pantry:

- Olive oil (best for salads and light cooking)
- Raw virgin coconut oil (best for strong heating)
- Sesame oil (good for heating)
- Hemp oil (dressings and dips; a long Russian and eastern Europe tradition)

Here are a couple more that are getting good reports:

- Palm oil (use the oil from the plant, not the kernel)
- Flax (too new to know whether this is a good prepared oil)

Last note on fats: you will notice a lack of mention of animal fats here, such as fish oils, butter, tallow, lard, cheese, ghee, and other dairy foods. While each of these may play a role in human diets, and even human health, they are specifically left out of a cleansing period, if for no other reason that to give the body a break. Few Westerners have ever gone one entire month (or two or six or twelve months) without animal foods and fats. Given that most people are doing a cleansing program in order to get rid of a health problem, it is always a good idea to "stop doing what you were doing, and do something else" during a cleansing period. If there is a need for fish or lean meats, use them as described in the section on animal foods. Other than that, use only plant-based fats.

❖ NUTS & SEEDS

Nuts and seeds are probably the best source for natural oil during an internal cleanse. They completely avoid the oxidation problems associated with turning nuts into liquid oils. They are also rich in vitamins (especially E) and minerals (especially magnesium, potassium, and copper).

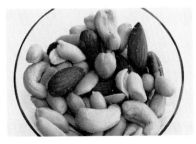

Because of their richness, think of nuts and seeds as a condiment, something to be sprinkled into a dish. Small amounts go a long way. As seductive as they are, moderation is the key when eating nuts and seeds. As you will see, once you start preparing the delicious cleansing recipes in the book, nut butters play a big role in sauces, both cold and hot.

Almost any nut or seed is fine. The main caution would be around peanuts, which are not really nuts, but legumes. Many people find them difficult to digest. In Indian Ayurvedic writings, peanuts are said to cause sluggishness and lethargy.

RAW, SPROUTED OR ROASTED?

While raw-food proponents like their nuts and seeds raw or sprouted, some people find that light roasting helps digest them. Nuts often have enzyme inhibitors that can be greatly reduced or nullified through a light roasting, soaking overnight, or sprouting. Like other dietary arguments, you are going to have to experiment with your own body and see what works for you.

Here are some of the nuts and seeds to have in your pantry:

- Seeds: sunflower, pumpkin and sesame
- Nuts and nut butters: almonds, walnuts, and cashews

❖ FERMENTED FOODS

Fermented, unpasteurized cultured foods are one of the real hidden secrets to good health. Ranging from vegetable dishes (sauerkraut, kimchi) to beans (tempeh, miso) and dairy (kefir), they all serve one purpose: to create a growing medium in which gut-friendly bacteria can thrive. In my experience, a solid month of eating 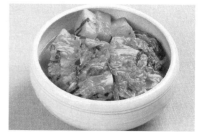 a cup of homemade fermented foods each day can turn around a broken digestive system. This is because when we prepare and eat them, we restock our digestive tract with the critical friendly flora that can so easily be killed with modern living.

In America, we do the strangest thing to our fermented foods: we pasteurize them. This kills all bacteria and enzymatic action, nullifying their effects. Few people have ever eaten a pickle that was actually enzymatically active. So, the best way to get powerful cultured vegetables is to make them yourself. It's really easy, almost mindless, and each batch gets better and better, because you keep a small portion of the last batch and mix it in with the next one. This matures the starter and speeds up the fermenting process. We have included a few fermented food recipes to get you started.

In the mean time, there are still a few products sold that are generally unpasteurized. In each case, you have to make sure that the brand you are getting did not heat treat them. You will have to ask. Here are some items that can come unpasteurized and can be part of your growing pantry:

- Olives (traditionally fermented, NOT heat treated)
- Umeboshi plums, paste, and vinegar
- Pickled ginger
- Salt-cured capers
- Shoyu or Tamari soy sauce
- Pickled vegetables, unpasteurized (see Sources section for manufacturers)
- Tempeh (a fermented soy product, see below)
- Miso

If the pickles you find have vinegar in the ingredients, it's not what you want. When vinegar is used to pickle, you can be sure that the food was heat treated, therefore destroying the enzymes and probiotics.

Naturally fermented foods made with Celtic sea salt and additions like spices, herbs, and garlic help make meals more digestible, promote the growth of healthy bacteria in the intestines (remember the 3rd R: rebacterialize), scavenge free radicals, make you less susceptible to yeast infections and Candida, help control diarrhea, dysentery, and assist the immune system. Many even say that it helps calm down their sweet tooth.

The bacteria in cultured foods facilitate the synthesis of vitamins, to the point where sauerkraut can have *a higher level of vitamin C than the raw cabbage from which it is made.*

Choline and acetylcholine are by-products of the fermentation. Choline helps us digest fat and decrease blood pressure. Acetylcholine is one of our body's most potent neurotransmitters, helping our parasympathetic nervous system digest and absorb food and regulate internal temperature.

Last interesting note on cultured foods: fermentation can reduce the amount of naturally occurring anti-nutritional components of vegetables. It can reduce nitrates in cabbage by over 80%, and reduce oxalic acid in beets by over 70%.

TEMPEH

Although not a common item in most households in the United States, tempeh has been a staple in Indonesia for over 400 years. It is made by cooking soybeans, adding a culturing agent, and then incubating the mixture overnight until it forms a solid cake. It is highly nutritious, one of the easiest beans to digest (because of the fermenting process), and makes one of the best substitutes for meat. Its distinctively nutty taste and texture easily absorbs the flavors of the other foods with which it is cooked making it adaptable to many types of dishes. Tempeh can be found in health-food stores and specialty markets throughout the year. If I were to eat only one bean dish, it would be tempeh.

MISO

Once you discover miso, you will wonder why you've never known more about it. As a live food, it is incredibly versatile. You can add it to soups, stews, guacamole, hummus, pesto, sauces, salad dressings, marinades and spreads to enhance digestion, help maintain a healthy cholesterol level and add essential amino acids and multiple complex B vitamins. The nutritional benefits of miso are outstanding and so is the taste.

Miso is low in fat, and rich in flavor. Like chicken or beef bouillon, it is used to add flavor to foods. Yet it is a much more functional food due to its beneficial microorganisms, lactobacilli and enzymes. The shelf life is very long, but it is best kept refrigerated or at least in a cool spot.

There are a variety of misos to choose from. Try the hearty barley and red misos for the root-vegetable and winter-squash dishes. The chickpea and light miso are perfect for spring and summer vegetables. You can blend different misos in your soups, and sauces. In the last few years, specialty misos have become available, such as the Garlic Red Pepper Miso from South River Miso

Co. The taste is so good, you can spread it thinly on Essene bread along with a bit of coconut or olive oil, or make a marinade for your salmon or mix it directly into rice.

Umeboshi plums, paste & vinegar

One of the most healing foods ever created is the umeboshi plum pickle, and the paste and salty brine products produced from it. It is largely unknown and unused in Western cultures, but it packs healing punch, as well as one of my favorite tastes. We use it daily in our meals.

Since at least the 1600s, this salty, tart pickled plum has been used as a cure for vomiting, intestinal worms, fevers, coughs and colds. The alkalinizing effects stimulate saliva and gastric juices, helping with the digestive process. The pyric acid helps with liver function and can help break down alcohol, probably the reason why umeboshi plums and tea are both suggested after a night of heavy eating or drinking. Umeboshi can be found as whole-plum pickles, pure paste (without the pit), and one of my favorites, umeboshi brine—found in stores as ume vinegar, but in fact it's just brine juice. As always, be sure you are getting true unadulterated, unpasteurized plums and plum products. The best and least inexpensive places to get large quantities are listed in the Sources section.

Last, there are two cultured food makers that I want to highlight. Mikala Moore, out of Durango, Colorado, has made some of the most delicious recipes I've tasted, and she has been kind enough to share some of her dishes here in the Recipes section. Also, check out the website of my friend Nancy Spahr, a colon hydrotherapist in Indiana, who is a cultured food expert:

www.cleansingwaters.info

She often has great recipes and ideas on her site.

The introduction of fermented foods to your diet can make one of the largest shifts this cleanse can offer. Refreshing, satisfying, and health-giving.

❖ SEA VEGETABLES

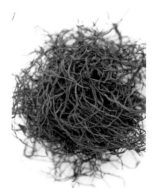

There is no better source of human-absorbable minerals than sea vegetables. From calcium, iron, zinc, and trace minerals, including iodine as well as vitamins A, B, C, D, E, nothing beats them for bio-availability. If you are reading this book because you want higher health, then you simply need to have a stock of sea vegetables in your pantry, and learn to cook them in mouth-watering ways.

Look at the impressive benefits: The brown algae family (Wakame, arame, kombu, and hijiki) will bind and expel radioactive substances and heavy metals from your body. They have a calming effect on moods. They balance hormones, reduce water retention and alkalynize the blood. They aid in digestion (all of our bean recipes include a piece of kombu). They are low in fat, high in fiber, and rich in the trace minerals that are often the key to turning around a health problem.

Find your entry level. For some it is the nori sushi wrap, or maybe the great seasonings available that combine ground up dulse or kelp and sea salt. After that, the step to arame and sea palm are short and oh so tasty.

For your pantry, start with:

Arame: mild, sweet and cooks quickly. It works well as a topping but also loves to be mixed with vegetables and grain dishes.

Hijiki: the best non-dairy source of calcium known. It has a strong flavor and likes to be mixed with other strong flavors such as, garlic, ginger, olives and tamari. Try marinating it before adding to salads, and vegetable dishes.

Kombu: mild taste and excellent for soups, stews and to cook with beans for extra digestibility.

Nori: the great sushi wrapper. It is ready to use so try it chopped into salads or cut in strips to use as crackers, Surprisingly, kids will eat this cut into squares and strips. They must know something! A friend of mine, Professor Steve Ottersberg, MS, toasts entire nori sheets by waving the 8-inch pieces over an open flame for about 2 seconds on each side, and then using them as a sort of catch all for anything you want to grab with your hands. Just plain delicious.

Wakame: is often used in miso soup. It has more of a sweet taste and is tender in texture, so it will break apart nicely in soups and stews. It is sometimes called Alaria, which is a version found in the Atlantic ocean.

Sea Palm: probably my favorite seaweed for taste and texture. If you're just starting out, try this one first. It has a nice subtle flavor and works well with salty, sweet and spicy flavors. Try toasting it and mixing it with tamari almonds for a quick snack. When it's soaked, it looks like pasta and is a refreshing alternative to it.

Wild Blue Green Algae: I've eaten a wild strain of fresh water algae (*Aphanizomenon flos-aqua*) daily for over 20 years. With lots of chlorophyll and its wide spectrum of trace minerals, it is, in my experience, one of the most powerful plants on earth. While you can't cook with it, you can use it as an encapsulated supplement, especially during a cleansing and healing period.

❖ BEVERAGES

Pure Water. During a cleanse, you want to be flushing your cells with plenty of water. A good rule of thumb is to take your total body weight, divide it in half, and then drink that amount in ounces. For example, if you weigh 100 pounds, drink 50 ounces of pure water. Do not use tap water. Get a filter, or purchase five-gallon containers of spring water. While distilled water may have its place in healing, stick with filtered or deep well spring water for its balanced minerals.

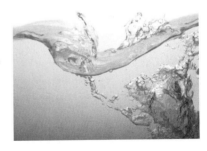

Herbal teas now come in hundreds of varieties. They are a great way to keep hydrated, and for those trying to lose weight, they help keep the digestive tract busy enough to avoid hunger. Use hot teas in the cooler months, and iced or chilled teas in the summer. Two naturally caffeinated herbal teas that work for many people are *herba matte* and green tea.

Fresh citrus coolers and teas are some of my favorite cleansing drinks. Simply squeeze lemons, limes, and oranges into cold or hot water. Sweeten with a teaspoon of honey, agave or maple syrup. To make your own gatorade-type drink, add a pinch of sea salt. I will often make a gallon at a time during the summer months. Lemons and limes are great liver decongestants.

Spritzers. If you are someone used to drinking cokes and sodas, you may miss that fizzy feeling. In that case, stock up on bubbly water, and flavor it with a bit of citrus or juice.

❖ CONDIMENTS & SEASONINGS

Here are the must haves:

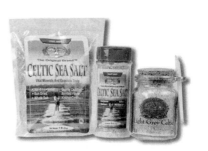

- Celtic sea salt
- Miso: a dark and a light version
- Olives, naturally fermented
- Tamari or Shoyu (two varieties of naturally fermented soy sauce)
- Umeboshi plums, paste, and vinegar (see Fermented Foods section)
- Apple cider vinegar (raw and unfiltered)
- Citrus fruit: lemons and limes to accent many dishes

These are optional:

- Mirin (a sweet fermented wine)
- Dried bonito fish flakes
- Hot sauces

❖ HERBS & SPICES

Adding various herbs and spices will not only enhance flavor but increase your body's ability to digest more efficiently.

For freshness, try to always have on hand ginger root and parsley. Both are considered to be a universal medicine and detoxifier.

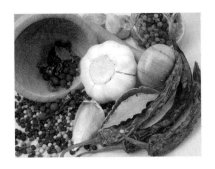

Some other spices:

- Cumin, cinnamon, coriander, chili powder, mustard seed, turmeric
- Basil, dill, rosemary, mint, sage, Herbs De Provence
- Dried hot peppers (all varieties)

Turmeric and ginger both assist in the digestion of protein (turmeric is actually a type of ginger).

Constipation & sluggish digestion: Cinnamon, fennel, marjoram, nutmeg, orange, black pepper, tarragon, turmeric

Heartburn: Cardamom, black pepper

Indigestion/ Flatulence: anise seed, lemon balm, basil, bay, caraway, cardamom, cinnamon, celery seed, clove, coriander, cumin, dill ,fennel, ginger, lavender, lemon, lemon grass, mandarin, marjoram, mint, nutmeg, orange, parsley, black pepper, rosemary, tarragon, thyme

Liver Congestion: Celery seed, rosemary, sage, turmeric, lemon

Loss of appetite: Bay, caraway, cardamom, ginger, black pepper

Curry: nine standard ingredients of curry include, turmeric, ginger, cardamom, coriander, cumin, nutmeg, cloves, pepper, and cinnamon

Herbs de Provence: any combination of 5 of the herbs listed here will work beautifully together: marjoram, thyme, summer savory, basil, rosemary, fennel seeds, sage and lavender

❖ Fruits & Dried Fruits

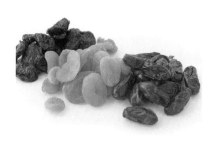

- Lemons & limes (try to always have a few on hand)
- Other citrus
- Apples, and whatever is in season
- Dried fruits, organic (avoid those that use preservatives or sugar)

Throughout the cleansing period, always have fresh fruit around. Try to eat fruit on its own, since if often causes gas and other digestive problems when eaten with grains, beans, and many vegetables. The rule of thumb is

1. Do not eat anything else for 60 minutes after eating fruit

2. Do not eat any fruit until 3 to 4 hours after your last meal.

In other words, let fruit digest on its own.

❖ Sweeteners

During a cleansing program, desserts and sweets need to be kept really simple. I often use nothing but fresh apples, or some sweetened tea after meals. And if you are dealing with some severe symptoms that have hounded you for years, this should probably be the extent of your sweets list.

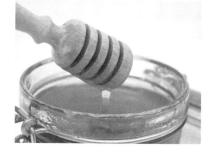

However, if you have had a lifestyle in which daily candy bars, ice cream, and plenty of sugar were the norm for the past few decades, you may find that you need to taper down a bit with some other quick energy dishes. Here are the sweeteners that are a easier on the system and that you can stock in your healthy pantry:

- Maple syrup

- Brown rice syrup
- Barley malt syrup
- Coconut milk, canned, no added sweeteners
- Mirin (a sweet rice vinegar)

There are some very effective tricks for weaning yourself off of a sugar-based diet:

Memorize this maxim: *if you are craving sugar, you are dehydrated.* Next time you go out to dinner, watch other diners and notice an interesting phenomenon: within 30-60 seconds of their last bite of their meal, most of them will crave a dessert. This rapid need for sugar is largely due to the dehydrating effect of a thick, hard-to-digest meal, especially if they have not drunk enough pure water during the day.

Before succumbing to the urge and subjecting yourself to a full-body sugar rush, be sure you are practicing good rehydration each day (1/2 your body weight in ounces of water). Also, try some sweetened herbal tea after dinner, and between meals. This is much more gentle on the system than cookies and a pint of ice cream.

❖ FREEZER & PACKAGED & CANNED FOODS

There are very, very few prepackaged foods that will work during a cleanse. It is too easy for companies to add low-quality salt, low-quality oil, and processed sweeteners to their products. So, in general, stay away from them.

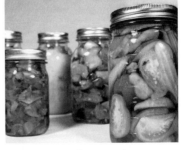

However, there are a growing number of conscious organic food companies offering clean, **single-ingredient** frozen, packaged, or canned foods that can have a place in your cleansing pantry. Just be very judicious with choosing and using them. **The rule of thumb is: one ingredient is best.**

FREEZER FOODS

For making fruit smoothies, soup broths, and the times when you are out of fresh vegetables, these are handy to have:

- Frozen organic peas, corn, and other vegetables
- Frozen organic 100% fruits (no sugar added)
- Frozen fish (for broths and stews)
- Frozen cranberries (these are a must, for their healing properties)

PACKAGED FOODS

- Organic soy milk (contains organic whole soy beans, salt, and water. Do NOT use the ones with sweeteners and oils)
- Rice or nut milk drinks
- Prepared mustard and hot sauces
- Tempeh (freezes very well)

CANNED FOODS

- Canned organic beans (whole beans, water, and salt)
- Canned organic coconut milk (coconut milk, and nothing else)

"Garlic is a powerful broad-spectrum antibiotic. It is also anti-viral, anti-fungal, anti-parasitic and has proven itself to rid the body internally and externally of any antigens or pathogens. Garlic has been used in hospitals and laboratories worldwide to destroy cancer and break up tumors, thin the blood and normalize blood pressure and cholesterol levels."

DR. RICHARD SCHULZE

❖ SUPERFOODS & THE "3 Rs"

In the book, *Cellular Cleansing Made Easy*, I went into great detail on the three most important missing ingredients of a modern day diet. They were friendly bacteria, trace minerals, and enzymes. Regaining them in one's daily fare was called getting "The Three Rs," which stands for ReMineralize, ReBacterialize and ReEnzymize.

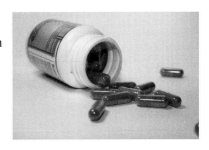

You can replenish these 3Rs through your diet, and you will be doing so by stocking your pantry and kitchen with the foods we suggest and by preparing the recipes in the "28-Day" section.

> You will **remineralize** by eating organic foods grown in deeply rich soil and using algae and other nutrient-dense foods.

> You will **rebacterialize** by eating foods that create an internal environment conducive to good bacteria, by eliminating processed sugars, and by daily consuming cultured vegetables, which contain billions of friendly bacteria (aka *flora*) in each tablespoon.

> You will **reenzymize** by eating raw foods, cultured vegetables, and drinking fresh vegetable juices.

Also, by eating foods with anti-fungal, anti-viral, and anti-parasite properties, your diet will start to take the place of the drugs and antibiotics that so many others use. While there are many foods that have these properties, we will focus mainly on the lowly garlic clove during the cleanse, since it is dirt cheap and so immediately and powerfully effective.

One of the other ways to speed up the healing and cleansing process is through superfood supplements. These guarantee that the necessary daily components get into us in concentrated amounts. Here are some suggestions:

- Probiotics (friendly bacteria). "wide spectrum" variety are best
- Blue Green Algae
- Herbal colon cleanse products
- Allimax™, an odorless encapsulated garlic with active *allicin*
- Clay (aka French, or Bentonite). Great intestinal detoxifier
- Spirulina or Chlorella
- Enzymes
- Green drink powders

❖ CRUNCH & ROAD FOOD

A cleansing diet doesn't include much of what could be called "crunch" foods— those crisp, loud, brittle foods and snacks that are so satisfying. While there are not any particular health advantages to crunch foods, there is an oral and sensation advantage, and some people crave them. If you are one of those people, there are some ways to keep crunch in your life.

- Carrot and celery sticks
- Baked mochi
- Nuts roasted in tamari
- Toasted Essene bread

One of the mistakes people make during a cleanse is not having any **road food** during their drive time. If you commute, or spend any amount of time in an automobile, you need to remember one warning: getting hungry while traveling is a recipe for disaster. Get a small cooler for the car, as a visual reminder to carry both snacks and water with you wherever you go. I *never* hop into my car without at least a jug of good water. Staying hydrated is a good way of avoiding an energy bonk when stuck in traffic. Fresh fruit is another.

❖ FOODS TO AVOID

During your cleanse, stay away from extremely processed and/or mucus-forming foods, such as:

- Dairy (milk, cheese, yogurt)
- Highly-processed fats & oils
- All power and protein bars
- Fake foods. Artificial anything
- Flour, processed flour products
- White, pasteurized vinegars
- Candy, soda, and sugared drinks
- Alcohol

Go easy on:

- Nightshades (see the section on Vegetables for more details)
- Caffeinated drinks and foods.
- Chocolate (see the section on chocolate under Food Controversies)

CHAPTER 7

Food confusions

One of the inescapable realizations that strikes anyone entering the world of the diet/disease, diet/symptom connection is that there are many viewpoints about what gets and keeps humans healthy. The world of nutrition is filled with conflicting debates about what is good, and what is not. These debates are affected by political, cultural, scientific, religious, ethical and even financial influences and beliefs. As both a student and a teacher, I can relate to the confusion that can come from this. But I want to suggest an alternative to confusion.

ADVOCATING EMPIRICISM

I would like to reintroduce an idea called empiricism. The concept of *empirical evidence* is an important one to any of us involved in the natural healing model. Empiricism loosely means *"evidence derived from personal experience."*

Why is this important? In a culture that generally only teaches, acknowledges and validates the scientific method of evidence, in which the only truth accepted is that concluded through laboratories, double-blind studies and lots of small rodents, empirical evidence allows each of us to be our own human laboratory, our own walking Petri dish. As the Internet becomes more and more of a giant Alexandria's Library, I believe that each of our empirical "hey, this is what happens to me when I do XYZ" communications are going to play a larger and larger role in how we determine what works and what doesn't. This sharing of experiences will not only help others in their search for healing, but will also be a powerful method for getting rid of dogmatic beliefs and this incessant and utterly ridiculous "I'm right, you're wrong" approach to health.

There are many other food confusions and controversies, but let's take a look at the few that will come into play during a cleansing program.

CARBO-PHOBIA

As this book is being written (the end of 2005), the Atkins Nutritionals corporation —one of the larger proponents of a fairly recent method of weight loss through carbohydrate elimination—has just filed for bankruptcy. Whether this signals a turn of the tide of what I call carbo-phobia isn't clear. But because of this weight-control system's popularity, and the public's general inability to make distinctions between white bread, soda pop, and whole grains grown in a farmer's soil, the following may be one of the more important parts to read in terms of your cleansing experience.

The essence of carbo-phobia is this: by starving the body of one of the essential building blocks of life, namely carbohydrates, the body starts to lose weight through a metabolic process called ketosis. Ketosis is a normal stage of metabolism that occurs any time the liver has been drained of glycogen (which has been derived from carbohydrates).

When people lose weight, they make an equation that translates something like this: "*Wow. Carbohydrates were my problem all along. I just proved it. Therefore carbohydrates are bad and I am not going to eat them.*"

The only reason a carbohydrate-free diet was ever invented was because 95% of the carbs consumed by people who gained weight came from extremely processed foods, such as soda, white bread, pasta, crackers, cakes, cookies, and sugar.

But there is a huge difference betwee these processed foods, and whole grains. One is good for you. The others are not so good for you.

Our body needs complex, full carbohydrates. It is in fact the only fuel the brain can use. Ask anyone that has gone on an Atkins diet and they will speak about the brain fog that occurred because of it.

Atkins and the other no-carb folks had it right in one aspect: stop eating processed carbohydrates. They're not good for you. They can clog up the system, wreak havoc with your blood sugars, and make it easy to gain weight.

But this all has little to do with the consumption of whole grains. So if you're suffering from carbo-phobia, it will help to have a perspective, and realize that long-living, healthy societies have used whole grains for centuries. You may just need a bit of faith with this cleansing program. Not only will you see changes, you will also feel them.

SOYBEANS

Since the 1970s, the U.S. has gone from using soybeans for feeding pigs, to soybeans for feeding people. In tofu, tempeh, tamari, and hundreds of protein powder drinks and bars, it became the savior food for a country questioning its animal treatment and animal consumption, and looking for a cheap source of protein.

In the last few years, the health benefits of soy have come into question. Since we have become a society that consumes more and more soy products, this can only be a good inquiry. However, most of the anti-soy articles and statements have been written in the panicked tone of Chicken Little's "The sky is falling."

The topic of soy, and whether it is *"good or bad for health because those are the only black and white choices right?"* is no different from questioning any other foods that we can place into our mouths in the form of nutrition. Humans have been doing this since the beginning of time. And what you learn is that foods are not necessarily 100% benign, or 100% poisonous. Some examples:

- Beets are one of the finest sources of Vitamin A and beta carotene. They're historically known as a blood purifier. But they also contain quite a bit of oxalic acid (especially the leaves) which is known to cause joint problems and kidney stones.

- All potatoes contain natural toxins called glycoalkaloids, usually at low levels. But higher levels of glycoalkaloids can be found in green parts of potatoes, sprouted potatoes and potatoes stored in light. Symptoms include headache, nausea, fatigue, vomiting, abdominal pain and diarrhea.

- Some foods do fine in animals, yet are harmful for humans (goats thrive on a type of thistle that is poisonous to people). The opposite is true as well: chocolate contains up to 2% theobromine, a psychoactive chemical that can kill a dog outright with as little as a half pound. If chocolate killed humans, my wife—and most women I've ever met—would have keeled over years ago.

There are scores of examples we could look at—from alcohol to celery to beef heart— all foods that are eaten and slurped every day by people who survive well into their old age.

Having been a big consumer of soy products since the late 70s, I have read these anti-soy articles with great interest. Although everyone should read their writings to make up their own mind, the essence of what they were saying is this:

- Soy beans are hard to digest. Further, if not prepared a particular way, they can block certain processes from happening inside the body.

- Much of the soy beans currently used have been genetically modified and are not the real deal.

- The large majority of soy-based products contain isolated soy proteins, from soy milk, to soy bars, to hundreds of other "hey-we're-vegeterian!" food products. Isolated soy protein should be treated no differently than white sugar and white flour. It's not the same as the whole bean.

- There are a growing number of symptoms that U.S. soy consumers are starting to see that may have a correlation to our soy consumption, such as B12 deficiency, pancreatic disorders, high levels of aluminum, and bone loss.

However, before you toss your tofu, consider this: some of the longest living people on earth use soy products, and have for hundreds of years. The inhabitants of the isolated Japanese island of Okinawa are regarded to be in the top three healthiest and longest-living peoples on earth. *"Scientists working for the U.S. National Institutes of Health and Japan's Ministry of Health have been following oldsters... since 1976 in the Okinawa Centenarian Study.... Elderly*

Okinawans tend to get plenty of physical and mental exercise. Their diets, more-over, are exemplary: low in fat and salt, and high in fruits and vegetables packed with fiber and antioxidant substances that protect against cancer, heart disease and stroke. They consume more soy than any other population on earth: 60-120 grams a day, compared to 30-50 grams for the average Japanese, 10 for Chinese and nearly 0 grams for the average American. Soy is rich in flavonoids—anti-oxidants strongly linked to low rates of cancer. This may be one of many reasons why the annual death rate from cancer in Okinawa is far below the U.S. rate."
(Time magazine, May, 2004, page 43, How to Live to be 100)

Highly processed foods are very different from their whole versions. Oki-nawans don't use soy milk, soy hotdogs, soy power bars or prepare their soy products in the historically new ways that we do. However, they are living lon-ger than any of us Westerners (Europe or the U.S.), and are therefore worth modeling. I think they're onto something.

Joann and I think soy products made from whole soy beans are good for you. And tempeh (a partially cooked fermented cake made from whole soybeans) is about the best way to use whole soy beans, so you'll find a few tempeh reci-pes throughout the program.

CHOCOLATE

Let's make a distinction: there is choco-late, and then there is cocoa. Chocolate is the combination of fat, sugar, and finely ground cocoa bean powder. Cocoa is just that finely ground dried powder from the bean of the cacao tree.

"I will never follow any diet that does not include chocolate."

ELIZABETH CORLEY,
FRIEND OF SCOTT'S

During a cleanse, you want to avoid any combination of fat and sweetener; there is probably no more insulting mixture when it comes to sludging up ones internal terrain.

Current nutritional literature is filled with information on the healthful effects of the cocoa bean. Flavanoids in it have been found to work as a mild anti-depressant. One of the body's chemicals produced during and after making love is *phenyl ethylamine,* and this is found in cocoa beans. Cocoa also helps release serotonin, a neurotrasmitter that is said to play a role in preventing depression and increasing sexual appetite.

Given the power of this simple, roasted bean in helping improve people's feel-good moods, it does not have to be off-limits during a cleanse. If you have found chocolate helpful in any of these ways, here is the cleansing rule: no more chocolate bars. Instead, get some of the new organic cocoa powder currently on the market and learn to make a simple hot water (or rice milk) and cocoa powder drink. Think simple *cocoa tea*, not chocolate bars, and you will still get the effects of chocolate without sludging up your cells.

SUNLIGHT & CANCER

Currently, one of the strongest beliefs out there is that exposure to the sun can cause skin cancer.

Here is another perspective: the skin is our largest elimination organ. Those who eat a diet rich in refined foods, refined fats, and chemicals, as well as using artificial soaps, scents, and shampoos are going to have the largest amount of metabolic waste coming out of their skin. It makes sense, then, that Westerners are seeing a huge increase in skin and sun related problems. Day in and day out, the sun reacts against this gunk coming out of the pores of the skin.

To add insult to injury, skin suffering from large amounts of metabolic waste can get dry and problematic. The current answer to this is to slather on gobs of skin creams because these products temporarily get rid of dryness, or makes it less wrinkly. Yet whatever is inside of those skin products gets absorbed into the deeper layers of the skin, and even into the blood stream.

Processed foods and many skin products are daily adding to the toxic load of your body. You have to question whether or not these substances are what the sun is reacting against.

The steadiest and most common change that people report when eating a cleansing diet, is that their skin improves. I have heard this daily for 20 years, and hear it all the time on the HowHealthWorks forum. What people are really saying is this: "My body's largest elimination organ has finally breathing and working the way it was designed to."

This has lead to an absurd paranoia of our sun. People cover up their body with clothes, and smear their largest breathing and absorbing and eliminating organ with substances (sunscreen), all under the illusion that this is the key to preventing a reaction on the surface of their body (called cancer) from occurring. This is like putting a cork in ones anus and hoping nothing comes out.

We need the sun. Lack of it is now being tied to hypertension, obesity, thyroid problems, arthritis, diabetes, heart disease, osteoporosis, fibromyalgia, and seasonal-affected disorder.

OTHER QUESTIONS & CONCERNS

Scott, you and Joann are not doctors.

I have always had two responses to this:

1. What does being an AMA medical doctor have to do with living a pharmaceutical-free life? It's almost a contradiction in terms. And,

2. Neither are you a doctor (most likely) but by the end of this program you will know more about the cause of skin and digestive injury, and what to do to repair it, than your doctor does.

This is not an exaggeration. No university—at least in America— currently teaches their medical students the diet/disease, diet/symptom connection as it relates to the many symptoms listed at the start of this book. This means that out of the 800,000 active medical doctors in the U.S., the large majority of them don't acknowledge this connection. They don't believe it. And, most importantly, they have not experienced this connection in their own body. Worse, they ignore the growing number of empirical examples of people who prove that Crohn's is a very curable symptom, that the answer to gallstones is a change in diet (not the removal of the gallbladder), and that psoriasis disappears once the liver is cleansed. The number of classically trained M.D.s that fully understand the diet-symptom connection is probably fewer than 100, and every time we hear of one, or read about one, we list them in our Resources section at HowHealthWorks.com. If you are an M.D. practicing and teaching these concepts, please let us know so we can list you in this online Resources section. The world needs to know about you.

When it comes to traumatic injury—broken bones, car wrecks, surgery, repairing eyes — I am grateful beyond words for the skills and the technology of our modern medical system. It is the M.D.'s realm of genius. But until our medical community heals itself of its unholy relationship to the pharmaceutical industry, and starts to treat the body the way a gardener views the soil, and they can point to any of those symptoms listed on the opening page and tell their clients, "Those are caused by what you have been eating," then those titled as a Medical Doctor will not be your best source for information on how to regenerate your body back to health.

I don't have time to eat like this.

Then you have not accurately done the math equation in two areas of life: one, how much your symptoms really cost you; and two, how much your sickness really costs your country's health-care system.

Saying you don't have enough time to eat a healing diet is like saying you don't have enough time to brush your teeth, or educate your children, or exercise. Our nation can no longer afford to ignore the skills of feeding ourselves as if our health depended on it. The marketing geniuses of the last 50 years has duped us into believing that we can live without real food (better living through chemistry and convenience). The truth is: if you rely on processed foods, eventually you will pay a heavy, heavy price.

I can't afford health food.

If you can afford to eat at McDonald's, and order pizza to go, then you most certainly can afford a cleansing-food lifestyle.

I don't know how to cook.

Neither did I when I first started. Learning to cook is like learning to type: it takes about five weeks of daily practice to not only create a healthy habit, but get skilled enough to feel comfortable. If you absolutely can't cook, then you will need to get a roommate who does, hire a cook, or live close enough to a health food store with a deli that prepares cleansing foods.

Healthy food tastes bland.

You can only say that because you've eaten bad-tasting health food, or you've never come over to Joann or Scott's house for lunch. The recipes in this book may have a cleansing effect on the body, but the truth is that they are so tasty, you'll want to eat this way all of the time.

One of the most-common results of cleansing is that people report an increased sensitivity in their taste buds. Once you move away from a diet rich in sugars, heavy fat and processing, a layer of sludge gets removed and food comes alive. Instead of a soup having one flavor, it has ten.

Cleansing is hard.

Compared to what? Really, ask yourself what you are comparing it to?

To me, "hard" is living with disease, or living with pharmaceutical drugs that are toxic to your body and that you know are not the real answer. "Hard" is believing that you don't have enough will power to change a few food habits.

One of the surest ways to increase your sense of self-esteem and well being is to dissolve habits that are bad for you, and replace them with habits that are life-enhancing. This takes two to four weeks. You can do this.

I can't afford organic food

That's fine. Use the cleanest foods you can find and afford.

Can I ever return to eating what I used to?

Well, first, you can eat anything you want. You always have been able to, and you always will be able to.

I think the real question is, "Once I've gotten rid of my symptoms through a cleansing diet, can I ever return to eating whatever I want without my symptoms coming back?"

Yes and no. Once a body heals deeply, and a strong immune system is in place, I find that people with digestion or skin problems can eat some of their former meals and drinks without getting symptoms. They just can't do it all the time. The occasional night of partying can be handled. Your skin will quickly tell you when enough is enough. For instance, let's say you have acne. In most cases, you will be acne-free inside of the first 40 days. At some point, you'll find you can occasionally eat the foods that helped create the internal condition that forced the skin to discharge as acne. Again, you just can't eat them very often.

Here is an analogy that may help. If you get injured playing a sport you love, there's no way you can return the next day and play the way you normally play. You have to go through a period of healing. The length of healing time will depend on the injury. Cut a finger? Take a day or two off. Bruise a calf muscle? Might take a week or two. Twist an ankle? It took me six months one time when I tripped over my dog's toy in the back yard while running from the sauna to the house (midwinter—I was in a hurry). Break a bone? You could be out for a year, and during that year, you have to stay within a narrow range of physical behaviors in order to not re-damage yourself.

The purpose of this book is not to makes foods wrong or right. It is to show how your food choices are deeply connected to your current state of health and your current list of symptoms. Cleansing shows us the cause and effect relationship we have—and always will have—with food and our health.

"In my many years of practice I have seen tens of thousands of patients recover from any and all disease using natural cleansing. Many people think that their particular disease or illness is unique. You may think that you are an exception. You are NOT. I have seen people sicker than you, people at death's door, people who all the doctors said would be dead a year before I ever met them. I assure you: I have treated people with every illness known, and everyone got well, as long as they did the work.

"I cannot get anyone well. I am a teacher. I can show you the path to great health, energy and vitality. I can take you on an adventure to a new life free of illness and pain. I can show you how to live longer and enjoy health beyond your wildest imagination. But you have to do the work. You are the one in control of your future health."

DR. RICHARD SCHULZE,
WORLD RENOWNED CLEANSING PRACTITIONER AND AUTHOR

PART TWO

RECIPES

Recipes

RECIPE CATEGORIES

➤ JUICES & RAW SOUPS

➤ GRAINS & GRAIN BOWLS

➤ BEANS & BEAN PRODUCTS

➤ SOUPS & STEWS

➤ VEGETABLES DISHES

➤ SAUCES & DRESSINGS

➤ FERMENTED FOODS

➤ SALADS

➤ QUICK ENERGY FOODS & DESSERTS

➤ SNACKS & CRUNCH

➤ DRINKS

Tips & Tricks

Pre-wash all your vegetables before you put them away is a great timesaver. You will like this especially when you go to make a juice. Wash your lettuce just after you buy it; then you'll have it on hand for salads when you need it.

Make large enough quantities to have leftovers. This is the biggest time saving tip of any cook, and you'll find that leftovers are often better tasting and can make the perfect base for a soup or topping for a salad the next day.

The Five Tastes: the Four Ss and One B. Always keep in mind the five main flavors. Try to have all five at least once per day:

- Sweet
- Sour
- Salty
- Spicy (aka pungent)
- Bitter

Make big quantities of all your grains and most beans; then you can prepare things quickly. Freezing small quantities of beans is a life saver on busy days. They're easy to thaw and are a cost cutting alternative to canned beans.

Learn all the tricks about making whole beans and whole grains digestible. See the earlier sections on these.

Find the dishes that are so simple to make, and so delicious to eat, that you can make and use them all the time.

A long list of ingredients does not mean that it is a labor intensive recipe. It simply means there are more complex flavors to experience. If you get everything out and even chop all your vegetables and measure your ingredients out before you turn on the heat, the payoffs of feeling organized and ready will boost the ease of cooking.

Keep your knife sharp! Purchase a knife sharpening steel, and do a few strokes each and every time you prepare a meal. Takes all of 15 seconds, and makes a big difference in the pleasure of cutting food.

If you're simply not in the mood for all those ingredients of a particular recipe, just cook with the basics. Olive oil, Celtic sea salt and the main vegetable or grain—with these simple items, you can never go wrong.

Read through the recipe twice to get the steps in your head. You'll notice how much smoother your cooking will go.

Some of these recipes will take you under 10 minutes to prepare. Use those when you're in a hurry. Learning to prepare food because you want to be able to serve quality meals in a short period of time is not a hard thing to accomplish.

If you are new to all of this, or new to cooking actual meals (instead of mainly prepared foods), just be patient. It usually feels awkward at first. Just know that every day you are learning the art of cleansing, you are adding to your skill level and knowledge.

Think differently. For instance, breakfast doesn't have to be sweet, made with something that spikes our insulin levels. It is actually quite satisfying and normal in some parts of the world for it to be savory.

For lunch, think leftovers, salads, soup. Make something to go or plan to go places where you can eat the foods available, such as salads, soups, hot grains and beans. Pack up some of last night's leftovers, add some fresh cut vegetables and sprouts with a great sauce you've pre-made and you've got an easy meal made in minutes.

Be prepared. When it comes to cleansing, the boy scout motto works well. Think ahead, and think about where you are going to get your food. If you work in an office, you need to remap where you will get nourishment. If you are driving, you need to have water and something to eat with you. Cleansing takes discipline and preparation and forethought.

If you're suddenly bored with your diet, change something. Try roasting or steaming or sautéing or pressure cooking or grilling or eating it raw. Do something different.

Some people love to cook, but who do you know who likes to cook every day, three meals a day? The key to better eating, is to find a way to make meals work for you instead of it making you crazy. Become a prep master. Having foods prepared in your fridge, freezer or pantry will help you be creative and less stressed out. One of my quickest meals is to open the fridge and look for 3 things: what greens do I have, what grain is cooked and what protein is there to add to them? Then I make a sauce to work with those three main parts and add the extras like sprouts and seeds for a little vitality.

Think quality. If a recipe calls for water, it means the highest quality water you can get, not tap water. If a recipe calls for salt, it means specifically whole Celtic gray sea salt, not enriched white salt that pours from its container. If it calls for garlic, it means fresh cloves. If it calls for herbs, try to use fresh, but dried will work just fine (generally about 1/2 of the fresh amount). It if calls for olive oil, use only extra virgin olive oil.

In other words, try to use the highest and purest source of ingredients you can find. Don't fret if you can't always get fresh or organic (none of us can). Just stock and use the best you can get.

Be flexible. If you see a recipe that calls for lemons, and you don't have any, try an orange, or a lime. If you don't have those, try making the dish without it. If the recipes calls for white beans, and you only have black, use those. If it asks for sage, and you only have thyme, use that. If the recipe contains tomatoes, and you're not suppose to use tomatoes, then prepare the meal without them. If it calls for 2 teaspoons of miso, and that turns out to be too salty, then use less next time.

In other words, cooking isn't an exact science. It's an art form, and like art, there are thousands of variations. Don't be afraid to play around.

"Before eating, always take time to thank the food."

ARAPAHO INDIAN SAYING

➤ JUICES & RAW SOUPS

During your cleansing program, you want to drink some fresh vegetable every day, anywhere between 12 and 32 ounces. Why? Juicing's biggest health benefit can be summarized in one phrase: cellular cleansing. Juicing works so well at cell cleansing because of a few reasons:

1. There is hardly any digestive work needed to process raw, enzymatically active liquid. Vegetable juice gets into the system quickly.

2. Squeezed vegetable juice is very nutrient-dense. This concentration acts to supercharge the system in the same way that herbal tinctures work.

3. Chlorophyll, a substance found exclusively in plants, has a structure similar to hemoglobin, the substance in blood that is responsible for transporting oxygen. During the 1940s, researchers found that consuming chlorophyll (all edible algae are rich in it) enhances the body's ability to produce hemoglobin, thus improving the efficiency of oxygen transport.

Enzymes are your body's work force. Acting as catalysts in hundreds of thousands of chemical reactions that take place throughout the body, enzymes are essential for digestion and absorption of food, for conversion of food stuffs into body tissue, and for the production of energy at the cellular level. In fact, enzymes are critical for most of the metabolic activities taking place in your body every second of every day.

Fresh juices are a tremendous source of enzymes, but they are destroyed by heat. If the food is cooked at temperatures above 114 degrees, the enzymes have been destroyed by the heat. Since fruits and vegetables are juiced raw, the enzymes are still viable when you drink the juice.

QUICK SQUEEZE HISTORY

Squeezing the liquid from plants is as old as agriculture itself, but it wasn't until the first quarter of the 20th century that juicing started to become popular as a tool for improving health. This came about largely because of two converging forces: the growing popularity of the Naturopathic and Natural Hygiene movements (both which were seeing results with fresh vegetable juicing), and a couple of timely technologies: refrigeration and juice extractors.

The first home juice extractor was not invented until the 1930s. It was called the Norwalk Juicer, by nutritionist Dr. Norman Walker. Walker was a fascinating thinker and health practitioner, on the same par as many of my own early health teachers. His exact age isn't known, but he was purportedly well over 100 years old when he finally died in 1984. His juicer worked by grating produce, placing the resulting mash in a bag, and then squeezing the bag under a hydraulic press. It was big and clunky, but it made great juice, and much of Walker's first books were filled with testimonies.

The next big innovation came in 1955 with the Champion juicer. The Champion was the first to pioneer the idea of forcing the pulp through a screen during the grating process. This shrunk the juicer down to kitchen counter size. From that point on, the juice extraction business exploded. Manufacturers started coming up with hundreds of models, trying different modes of extraction, and becoming smaller and easier to use over time. With ease and availability, tens of thousands of consumers purchased juicers and started adding to the pile of empirical evidence that showed the healing properties of juicing.

General Juicing Tips

In general, make your juice taste good.
I divide vegetable juices into two categories: Delicious juice, and Tequila juice. **Delicious juice** is the kind that you drink and immediately think "ahhh!" You could drink a quart a day, even your UPS driver would like it, and it's generally enjoyed any time. **Tequila juice** is the kind of medicinal juice that you sip and immediately make a face. This is the intensely green drink, the kind that immediately opens up every duct in your gall bladder and liver. I call it this name because it's best done in small 1 to 4 ounce amounts, shot back like you would with tequila, and works best if you finish with a grimace, a grin, and a loud "Yeah!" Try a little of both kinds each week.

Easy on the fruit
I am not a big fan of using my juicer to make and consume 100% fruit juices.

Fruit is great, one of best quick energy sources and can be very healing in its own way, but I would suggest just eating an apple or orange.

That said, don't be afraid to add some citrus, rind and all. Or half an apple, a few grapes, or a handful of cranberries. A bit of lemon and lime actually do quite well when combined with most vegetables. I've also found this true with apples and cranberries.

To avoid clogging the screens and having to clean them mid-juicing, alternate your soft and hard produce. This will help clear out the screens. Done right, I can juice a full quart without having to stop and clean the screen.

The "baseline" vegetables: carrots, parsnips, cabbage, beets, celery, cucumbers, broccoli, burdock root...

The bitter greens: kale, collards, parsley, wheatgrass, lettuces, dandelion, watercress...

The "high note" vegetables: Caution! With the exception of ginger, use very little of these: onions, ginger, radish, chives...

The "high note" fruits: apples, lemons, limes, oranges, cranberries, grapes...

I don't think it is necessary to get too specific about which juice works best for each condition and symptom. I would just start juicing. Still, it's interesting to note that every vegetable has its own particular healing properties.

> **Cucumber** juice is thought to clean your kidneys, lower high blood pressure and improve skin problems (I've found this skin part to be especially true).

> **Cabbage** juice is one of the most healing nutrients for stomach repair. Contains sulfur and selenium, both which are good for joint stiffness. While cooked cabbage can give me gas (ask my wife), I digest raw cabbage with no problem.

> **Beets** are famous for their ability to cleanse the blood and strengthen the gall bladder and liver. Beet juice is very concentrated, so a little goes a long way; try 20% of the total amount.

> **Broccoli**: Even the staid National Cancer Institute is excited about this plant, saying that it's showing anti-cancer properties. A strong taste, so I only add about 10%.

Apples: I think tart apples are one of the most underrated healing foods we have. Apples contain malic acid, which is capable of softening gallstones and other calcifications in the body. In August, when organic, wild apples are falling off the trees around our Colorado county, I take that as a hint to clean out my liver. My wife and I will drive around and get a bushel of these amazing little apples and juice them up (it's one of the few times I drink 100% fruit juice). There are few things in life that make people roll their eyes up in ecstasy, and this apple juice we make is one of them. If there is a heaven, they serve it there.

Celery: long considered a nerve tonic.

Parsley: very high in chlorophyll.

Cranberries: Contains quercetin and tannins, flavonoids that are getting much attention for their anti-bacterial, inflammatory and tumor properties. They help to cleanse the kidneys by lowering uric acid levels (often associated with gout, kidney gravel, and joint pain). Cranberries are one of the few frozen foods I'll let into my juice, mainly because you can now find them raw and organic in the freezer section.

Collards and Kale have more calcium than milk, and in an extremely bio-available form.

If you do use fruit in your juice, especially apple, don't eat anything solid for 60-90 minutes afterwards, to prevent indigestion. Let the juice do its work by itself, so that it is the only thing in your digestive tract.

A pinch of Celtic gray sea salt can perk up many juices.

I often use fresh ginger root in juice, especially in combination with apple. Ginger helps lower nausea and inflammation, relieves pain, and aids with circulation.

Wheatgrass is an alkalinizing miracle unto itself, belonging to the "tequila juice" category. I always drink it separate from my other juice, and I always mix in a half lemon.

Joann and I often get people questioning if some vegetables are too high in natural sugar. I've seen people eat flour-based "health" desserts on a regular basis and then say they don't juice because it has "too much sugar." I'd suggest exactly the opposite. One evening, instead of eating flour products, try juicing before your dinner. I look forward to the day when our biggest health challenge is "too much carrot juice" coming from vending machines in our school cafeterias, versus soda and candy bars. "Did you hear what they're now serving in the vending machines at my kid's grade school? Fresh carrot and celery juice! That's way too much sugar for my kid! Yeah, I want them to go back to the Snicker's bars."

If your juice is too sweet for you, cut it in half with water. Don't be afraid of seeing how you respond to fresh enzymatic juice.

Don't be alarmed if you go through a bit of detoxification in the first couple weeks. That's normal and temporary, and the blessing of the plant kingdom.

While you can make fruit juice with your juicing machine, you are better off just eating a piece of fruit. It is too easy to drink down a couple pints of fresh fruit juice, which represents a few pounds of pears or grapes or whatever fruit you chose. While delicious, it can be more concentrated sweetness than is good for the body.

Store any extra juice in either an air tight glass container (if you plan on using it over the next couple of days), or by freezing it.

Make all your juice in the morning and have it to drink throughout the day-

Choose from these ingredients for juicing:

• Carrots	• Beets (small amounts are better)
• Celery	• Parsley, cilantro, dill, basil
• Cabbage	• Ginger
• Fennel	• Kale, dandelion, lettuces,
• Wheatgrass	• Sprouts
• Cucumber	• Radishes
• Tomatoes	• Apples
• Citrus: lemon, lime, orange	• Grapes
• Pineapple, grapefruit	

I never put garlic in my juice. I eat raw garlic all the time (there is no stronger anti-fungal/bacterial/viral food out there) and it's one of life's true super-foods, but I refuse to make my juices taste bad.

Squeezing vegetables isn't the Be All, End All to staying healthy. And it's not the main ingredient of this cleansing program. But it has helped me stay flexible and symptom-free for the past two decades.

JUICE RECIPES

Juicing with recipes is not necessary. To begin, start with equal parts of carrots, cucumber and celery. Add a piece of ginger and handful of parsley. Add 5% from the bitter green list. Add a piece of apple or citrus. That's about it.

However, if you want some ideas, try these:

Basic Daily Juice

• 1/3 carrot	• 1/3 cucumber
• 1/3 celery	• Ginger, small piece
• Leafy green or parsley, 5%	• Apple, small piece (optional)

Wheatgrass Hopper

• Juice 1 whole lemon	• 1 ounce of wheat grass juice
• fresh pineapple, 4-8 ounces	• fresh mint leaves

Green Power

• 3" of cucumber	• 1 stalk celery
• A few leaves of kale	• 1 inch ginger
• ½ fennel bulb	• ½ cup parsley

Green Tang

• Apple	• Kale
• Spinach	• Lime

Apple Carrot

• Carrot 8	• Apple 2
• Celery, 2 stalks	• Cabbage leaves, 2 or 3

Susan's Secret

• Celery	• Cabbage
• Cucumber	• Lime

Hit the Spot

• Carrot	• Ginger
• Apple	• Beet (small amount)

Broccoli Calcium Drink

• Celery	• Lemon
• Broccoli pieces	• Parsley (10%)

Cold Gazpacho

Gazpacho from a juicer is one of the most delicious, satisfying dishes I know, and I will often eat nothing but this for a few days during a cleansing phase. It is a very concentrated way to get nutrients into you, and it's very cooling on the liver and gallbladder. It's also very easy and quick to make, and can be done with any high end juicer.

Put the "blank" screen into your juicer, the one that allows everything (both pulp and the juice) to fall straight through into your bowl. There is no real recipe, other than to juice a quart of vegetables (juice and pulp) and then adjust the taste with lemon and sea salt. Here's a sample mix of vegetables to start with:

• Cucumber (30%)	• Zucchini (30%)
• Carrot (10%)	• Beet (10%)
• Tomato (just one or two)	• Lemon and salt to taste

For extra taste, add a tablespoon of dark sesame oil, or coconut oil. Other ingredients can include:

• Avocado (*delicious!*)	• Parsley, basil, cilantro
• Almonds (or Cashew Sour Cream)	• Black pepper
• Onion, garlic	

➤ GRAINS & GRAIN BOWLS

BASIC TIPS

Rinse grains thoroughly in cold water until the water turns clear (just use the pot that you are cooking in for this). Toss the rinse water and then add the cooking water. When the recommended time has gone by, test the grains to see if they are done (a slight chewy texture is good). One of the best tips I ever learned was from master chef Caroline Dino (who cooked at Scott's wedding): turn off the heat during the last 15 minutes, and cover the cooking pot with a thick cloth in order to keep the heat in. This keeps the cooking going, but prevents burning and makes for a fluffier grain.

Each grain has its own unique texture. Quinoa, wheat berries, and brown rice cook so that each grain is separate, so these are best used for grain dishes. Amaranth, whole oats, teff and millet make great porridge. Once the water is boiling, cover the pot, reduce the heat and simmer until the grains are soft. Don't lift the lid if you can help it; let the steam do its work.

Soaking grains before cooking. This method may seem odd, but it produces excellent results in digestibility and is key to absorption instead of blockage of nutrients from the grain. The high rates of sensitivity to proteins from grains create problems such as celiac disease, allergies, chronic indigestion and Candida. Soaking or simple fermentation will encourage the production of beneficial enzymes, lactobacilli and other helpful organisms to break down harmful nutrient inhibitors, which can lead to mineral deficiencies and even bone loss. Get into the habit of soaking your grains as well as your beans; your stomach and intestines will know the difference.

Toasting your grains before cooking adds flavor and digestibility. For variety, add seaweed, onions or other seasonings during the cooking.

Add a pinch of salt for every cup of dry grain. This goes for all grains.

How To Prepare Each Grain

Amaranth

Amaranth is a gluten-free ancient Aztec grain. It is a high quality protein and has 60 mg of calcium per ½ cup. It has a sticky, gelatinous-like texture more like porridge when cooked. Our favorite way of using it is to combine some with buckwheat, millet, or brown rice, or even as a thickener to stews. It can also be popped like corn.

- 1" piece of kombu (optional, but it adds minerals and digestibility)
- 1 cup grain to 2 ½ cups liquid
- Pinch of salt per cup of grain
- Simmer 20 minutes
- Yields 2 ½ cups cooked grain

Barley

Barley's chewy texture tastes delicious when mixed with other dishes. It has 50% percent more protein than wheat and more iron and calcium, too. Add it to stews and soups, combine it with other grains or cook in extra liquid to make a breakfast porridge.

- 1" piece of kombu (optional, but it adds minerals and digestibility)
- 1 cup grain to 3 cups of liquid
- Pinch of salt per cup of grain
- Simmer about 60 hours
- Yields 4 cups of cooked grain

In a heavy medium sized saucepan, put kombu, barley and water. Cover and bring to a boil over medium heat. Turn the heat down to low, add salt and cook for at least 60 minutes until barley has absorbed all the water.

Buckwheat (Raw or Toasted)

- 1 cup grain to 2 ½ cups liquid
- Pinch of salt per cup of grain
- Bring to boil, and simmer for 15-20 minutes

Roasted buckwheat is also called kasha. It has a stronger flavor and a drier texture than raw buckwheat. It is great in pilaf mixed with rice, veggies, garlic, and other seasonings.

Don't pressure cook buckwheat. It gets mushy too easily. To avoid mushiness, cook 1 cup roasted buckwheat with 1 beaten egg in a heavy saucepan over medium heat. Cook, stirring until dry. Add 2 cups boiling liquid. Cover, reduce heat and simmer 20 minutes. Fluff.

Job's Tears (aka Chinese Pearl Barley)

Job's tears have a long history for being a truly medicinal plant. Eastern medicine says that they are very helpful for removing excess water from the body, used as a tea for weight loss, helps with urinary infections, effective for loose bowels, and is included in many anti-tumor formulas.

- 1 cup of Job's tears to 2 cups of liquid
- Pinch of salt per cup of grain
- Bring to boil, simmer for 45 minutes

NOTE: Job's tears often seems to come with a few small similar-sized pebbles mixed in with it (Scott broke a tooth once eating Job's tears). Don't let this stop you from using this extremely healthful grain, but do be very careful in the cleaning and rinsing process.

Job's tears is also known as Chinese pearl barley; this is completely different than *pearled* barley, which is a processed form of barley that has had some of its nutrients removed. Don't confused the two.

Kamut

- 1" piece of kombu (optional, but it adds minerals and digestibility)
- 1 cup grain to 3 cups liquid
- Pinch of salt per cup of grain
- Simmer 2 hours

This is an ancient Egyptian wheat with a very chewy texture. Compared to regular wheat, it is 30% higher in protein and richer in vitamins and minerals. It does contain gluten, but many wheat-sensitive people can eat it without a problem. It is great hot or cold. Marinate it and add it to salads. Use it instead of rice.

Millet

Millet is considered one of the oldest grains, having been used for over 12,000 years. It is the main grain used by the Hunza tribe, which is famous for its healthy people. *Millet has more iron than any other grain in the world.* After you rinse it well, try toasting it before you add the water to cook. The aroma is wonderful and the natural nutty flavor comes out.

- 1" piece of kombu (optional, but it adds minerals and digestibility)
- Pinch of salt per cup of grain
- 1 cup millet to 4-5 cups of liquid

Bring millet and water to boil in a covered skillet or saucepan. Reduce the heat, cover and simmer for 20 minutes until all the liquid is absorbed. Then let sit covered for 20 minutes. Fluff up and serve.

Oat Groats

- 1 cup whole oat groats to 3 or 4 cups of water
- Simmer for 2 hours (or overnight)

Most people have never purchased or cooked whole oats, also called groats. Whole oat groats are the only way to go—you will see, taste, and even feel the difference. Do not use cut oats, rolled oats, or quick oats during your cleanse; they've been processed and have lost some of their nutrients, their digestibility, and the oils found in them are generally rancid or missing. If you presoak groats overnight, you can reduce the cooking time to 80 minutes. Or you can slow cook overnight in your crockpot for breakfast.

Overnight Oats:

- 2 cups oat groats, rinsed and soaked
- 6-8 cups water
- Pinch of salt per cup of grain

Rinse groats. Bring to boil. Add salt. Lower flame, put over a flame tamer (see Tools section) and cook overnight. You will not believe the amount of oat cream that rises to the top. This is one of Scott and Joann's favorite breakfasts. Try adding some dried fruit; it nearly melts and the flavor is delicious.

Quinoa

Quinoa (keen' wah) is a sweet grain this is chock full of nutrients, easy to digest and a great compliment to many other foods including other grains. There is no other grain that feels so light and has quite an interesting texture.

- 1" piece kombu (an option with any grain; adds minerals and digestibility)
- 1 cup quinoa, rinse and drain well.
- Pinch of salt per cup of grain
- 2 cups water

Rinse well. Bring water, quinoa and kombu to a boil in a saucepan, with a pinch of Celtic sea salt. After its comes to a boil, cover, reduce heat to low and cook for 20 minutes until all your water is absorbed.

Brown Rice

Pressured cooked rice

- 1 cup rice to 2 cups water (or a little less)
- 1 piece of kombu seaweed 3-4 inches long
- Pinch of salt per cup of grain

Put all in cooker and bring to a boil. Add Celtic sea salt, seal the pressure cooker with the top, and bring up to pressure. Once it is at full pressure, leave at high heat for 1 minute, then lower heat to a simmer. We prefer to use a flame tamer (aka a heat deflector) at this point. Cook for 45-50 minutes. We also like to keep it on the flame for 30 minutes, then remove and cover for the remaining time.

Nutty Stovetop Rice

- 1 cup of rice to 2 cups of water
- 2 ¼ cups of rice, use 4 cups of water
- 3 ½ cups of rice, use 6 cups of water
- Pinch of salt per cup of grain

Rinse the uncooked rice well, then drain. In a separate pan, boil the cooking water. While waiting for it to boil, put a couple tablespoons of olive or coconut oil in the bottom of a heavy, tight-lidded sauce pan, then sauté the well-drained rice in the oil. Do this over fairly high heat. It has to be stirred constantly, otherwise it will scorch. This process coats the rice with the oil and evaporates the water from rinsing. The rice will begin to smell very nutty after a minute or two.

When the water in the other pan has come to a vigorous boil, pour it over the rice in the sauce pan. It is very important at this point not to stir the rice anymore, not even once. Let it come back up to a vigorous boil, put the lid on, turn it down as low as you can and cook for 45 minutes. During this time, do not lift the lid or do anything else to it. When 45 minutes is up, turn off the heat and let the rice sit undisturbed for at least 15-20 minutes before serving.

WILD RICE

- Use 1 cup grain to 3 cups liquid
- Pinch of salt per cup of grain
- Bring to boil, then simmer 45-60 minutes (or just cook it with another grain)

Wild rice is actually not a grain, but a grass. It combines well with many other grains and vegetables. You can toss a handful in when cooking other grains.

Teff

Teff is an ancient grain that is finding a resurgence in the health food world. Its history goes back to about 3300 BC when it was the main grain of Ethiopia and India. It is now being grown in places like Idaho.

- Use 1 cup teff to 4-5 cups liquid
- Pinch of salt per cup of grain
- Boil, then lower the heat and simmer 20-25 minutes

Teff makes a brilliant morning porridge; use it in place of oats. But our favorite usage, just like Amaranth, is to mix about 10-20% with other grains for added flavor and texture.

Wheat Berries

Wheat is currently a word that makes many folks break out in hives the minute they see it in print. It is on many people's food phobia list because they know that wheat kernels (also known as wheat berries) are the original source of all of the processed sludge-producing bread, cakes, cookies and cold cereals that used to be daily eaten and has gummed up their inner works so severely that they now react to anything made from wheat flour. But like the difference between coca leaves and cocaine, or white crystalline sugar and a section of cane cut from the field, there is a large difference between a full 100% organic wheat berry, and the flour found in a bagel. And no, a "whole grain" muffin has very little to do with whole grain wheat berries. So, if you have never eaten a meal that uses wheat berries, give it a try.

- 1 cup wheat berries to 3 cups liquid
- Pinch of salt per cup of grain

If possible, soak the berries overnight. Boil water in a large saucepan, add wheat berries. Reduce heat to simmer, cover and cook until water is absorbed, about an hour.

Grain Dishes

Once you have your grains prepared and ready in the refrigerator, you'll be able to make great combinations with a variety of seasonings, vegetables and beans.

Quinoa with Jicama, Cilantro and Lime

• 1 cup quinoa, rinsed well	• 1 cup cilantro, chopped
• ½ cup celery, chopped	• Juice of 2 fresh limes
• ½ cup olives, chopped	• Olive oil

Rinse and drain quinoa well. Add to 2 cups of water in a saucepan and a 1" piece of kombu seaweed. Bring to a boil, add a pinch of Celtic sea salt. After its come to a boil, cover, reduce heat to low and cook for 20 minutes until all your water is absorbed. Let cool.

In a bowl, combine celery, jicama, cilantro and olives. Combine with quinoa, mixing gently. Dress with oil, lime, salt and pepper.

Millet Lentil Pilaf

This combination works well when the vegetables are chopped small.

• 1 cup millet, rinsed	• 4 tablespoon olive oil
• ½ cup each onion, carrot and celery, chopped	• ½ cup sunflower seeds, toasted and chopped
• ¼ cup fresh parsley, chopped	• ½ cup chopped mushrooms
• 1-2 tablespoon chopped olives	• 3 cups boiling water
• Celtic sea salt & fresh pepper	• ½ cup cooked lentils

First heat up 2 tablespoon of oil in a saucepan, add rinsed millet, a ½ teaspoon salt and heat until coated with oil and a nutty aroma comes out. Add 3 cups boiling water, turn heat down to simmer, cook for 35 minutes, covered.

In a skillet, heat 1 tablespoon oil, and sauté the vegetables for about 7-10 minutes on medium heat until they are soft. Lower heat, add sunflower seeds, millet and lentils until they are heated through. Add parsley and season with salt and pepper. Mix well. This dish tastes great served with sauerkraut.

Tabbouleh with Quinoa

This middle Eastern staple is especially good with quinoa replacing the usual bulgar wheat, which wouldn't work during a cleanse. And I like to keep the grain to a minimum, filling up on the parsley and vegetables instead.

• 6 cups fresh parsley, chopped	• ½ cup fresh mint chopped
• 6 scallions	• 6 tablespoon fresh lemon juice
• ½ cup cooked quinoa	• ½ teaspoon Celtic sea salt
• ¼ cup olive oil	

Add all ingredients to a bowl and adjust lemon, salt and pepper to taste.

Other optional ingredients are:

• 1 cucumber, diced	• ½ cup fresh mint chopped
• ½ cup red onion, chopped	• 1 cup cooked chickpeas

Wheat Berry Waldorf Salad

You can use lots of variations for this salad. Substitute dates, apricots or currants for the raisins; pine nuts or almonds instead of walnuts. Add oranges, or red peppers. It's a great way to eat the wheat berries and give them some snap.

• 4 cups water	• 1 cup wheat berries, rinsed
• 2 Granny Smith apples or other crispy tart variety, chopped	• 3 tablespoon apple cider vinegar (unpasteurized)
• ¼ cup raisins	• ¼ cup walnuts, toast & chop
• 1 carrot grated	• ¼ cup chopped mint leaves
• 3 tablespoon orange juice	• ½ teaspoon orange zest
• 1 stalk celery chopped	• Salt and pepper

Boil water in a large saucepan, add wheat berries and bring back to boil. Reduce heat to simmer, cover and cook until water is absorbed, about an hour. Spread the berries out to cool.

In a large bow, mix wheat berries, apples, celery, carrots, raisins, walnut and mint. In a small bowl, whisk together orange juice, zest and apple cider vinegar. Pour over grain mixture and season with salt and pepper. If necessary, add more apple cider vinegar and orange juice.

Coconut Rice

• 2 cups long grain brown rice	• 1 tablespoon coconut oil
• 1 can coconut milk (no sugar)	• 1 cup water
• 1 cinnamon stick	• ½ cup chopped cashews

Rinse rice thoroughly and drain. In a saucepan heat coconut oil on medium heat. Add rice and cook, stirring constantly until it becomes opaque, about 3 minutes. Stir in coconut milk, water, nuts, cinnamon and salt. Bring to a boil. Reduce heat to simmer, cover 20 minutes. Then remove from heat and let stand 5 more minutes. Remove cinnamon before serving.

Slow Cooker Mushroom Risotto with Peas

• ¼ cup dried porcini mushrooms	• 1 cup boiling water
• 3 tablespoon olive oil	• 2 shallots, minced
• 1 cup shiitake mushrooms	• 1 ¼ cups short grain brown rice
• 2 ½ cups vegetable broth	• 1 large garlic clove, minced
• 1 cup cremini mushrooms	• 2 teaspoon dried thyme
• 1 teaspoon salt	• 2 tablespoon tamari
• 1 tablespoon minced parsley	• Fresh ground pepper
• ½ bag of frozen peas	

Soak the dried porcini in boiling water for 30 minutes. Drain, reserving 3/4 cup of the liquid. Chop the mushrooms and set aside.

In a small skillet, heat oil over medium heat. Add the shallots and garlic, cook until slightly soft, about one minute. Transfer this to a 4 qt quart slow cooker. Add the rice, stirring to coat with the oil. Stir in all the mushrooms, the remaining reserved liquids, water, thyme, and salt. Cover and cook on high for about 1 1/2 hours, then add peas. Cover and finish cooking for another 1/2 hour, until all liquid is absorbed.

Just before serving, add fresh parsley, tamari and fresh pepper.

Millet Cauliflower Mash with Pesto

This dish is a prize among grain lovers. I've seen it very simply done, or with a bulb of fennel or cut up carrots cooked in it. It has been written up in so many healthy foods cookbooks but I had decided it needed a twist. This version is delicious and simple.

• 3 cups cauliflower, small pieces	• 1 cup millet
• 1 cup diced onion	• 3 cups water
• ¼ cup pesto	• 2 tablespoon light miso

Wash, drain and toast the millet in a skillet (skip this if you are short on time). Put all ingredients in pressure cooker, except miso and pesto. Bring to pressure-cook 20 minutes on low flame. Whip together. Add water if needed for a consistency of mashed potatoes. Add miso. Stir in pesto or serve on the side for guest's option.

Stir fried Rice

When you have rice or any grain already cooked, try stir-frying some vegetables and combining it all for a fast, delicious meal, breakfast, lunch or dinner. 2-3 cups precooked rice, cold from the refrigerator is best.

• 1 small onion or 4 scallions	• 1 cup carrot, chopped
• 1–2 tablespoon olive oil	• 1 tablespoon ginger, grated then squeezed for the juice
• 1-2 tablespoon tamari	

Other vegetables to use, but don't limit yourself:

• Mushrooms	• Jerusalem artichoke
• Green beans cut diagonally	• Mung Sprouts

Start by heating your oil in a wok or large skillet with medium to high heat. Then add your crunchy vegetables, like the carrots and cook for a few minutes. Add the onions and green beans, cook for another couple minutes. Add rice and tamari and heat thoroughly.

Savory Quinoa Pilaf with Pomegranates and Leeks

• 2 cups water	• 1 cup quinoa, rinsed well
• 1 cup leeks, chopped	• 1 tablespoon coconut oil
• ½ tsp salt	• ½ pecans, chopped
• ½ pomegranate	• 2 tablespoons fresh thyme

In a medium saucepan, bring water and quinoa to a boil. Reduce heat to simmer, cover for 20 minutes until all the water has been absorbed. Let cool. In another sauté pan, heat the olive oil and sauté the leeks until soft and golden. Remove from heat and stir into the cooled quinoa. Add nuts, pomegranate seeds and fresh thyme and a drizzle of olive oil. Season with salt and pepper.

Marinated Portobello with Barley Pilaf

First, make the Mushroom Marinade:

• 2 tablespoon dark miso	• 2 tablespoon balsamic vinegar
• 4 tablespoon water	• 3 tablespoon olive oil
• 2 tablespoon tamari	• 1 clove of garlic, minced
• 2 tablespoon chopped basil	• 4 whole Portobello mushrooms
• 6 scallions, sliced thin	

In a small bowl, whisk together the olive oil, miso, water, tamari , garlic and basil. Put the mushrooms in a larger bowl with a lid and pour the marinade over them, turning frequently for about 20 minutes.

Sauté the mushrooms on medium-low heat, whole in olive oil. Add scallions and let simmer on low-medium heat until the mushrooms are tender; about 20 minutes or more or less. If you keep the heat low, you will retain the nutritive integrity of the miso, but don't worry, even if the heat is high, you will still get great flavor from the marinade.

These mushrooms also work well on kabobs in the broiler or grill. You can cut them into 2-3" chunks and marinate along with zucchini, red pepper, tempeh and onions. The cooking time will be quicker though, 10 minutes at the most.

Serve over Barley Pilaf or quinoa with a side of salad greens. The natural combination of the rich mushrooms and hearty barley with the freshness of greens is a delightful surprise.

Barley Pilaf

• 1 cup barley, soaked	• ¼ cup onion, chopped
• ¼ cup mushrooms, chopped	• 2 cups water
• ½ teaspoon Celtic sea salt	• 1 teaspoon tamari

In a medium saucepan, sauté the onions and mushroom stems for 3 minutes. Add barley and continue to stir fry for another minute. Then add water or mushroom broth and simmer until liquid is absorbed, about 40-50 minutes. Serve pilaf with mushroom over fresh salad greens; arugula, dandelions or simple leaf lettuce all work well. Sprinkle with scallions and walnuts.

Breakfast Grains

Oat Cream

Soak 2 cups whole oat groats for 12-24 hours.

Stovetop oat cream version:

Rinse groats, add water to cover, a generous pinch of sea salt and bring to a boil. Reduce heat to low, cover and cook until done, they should be very tender and creamy (about 2 hours).

Slow cooker oat cream version:

• 2 cups oat groats	• 8 cups water
• Pinch of sea salt	

Rinse the grain. Cook overnight, using a low flame and a flame tamer (see the Tools chapter). Serve with maple syrup, raisins, coconut, chopped nuts, or dried fruits.

Creamy Rice Cereal

1 cup of short grain rice	4 cups water

Rinse and drain rice thoroughly 3 times. Add to water, bring to a boil, simmer for 75 minutes. Take off, then using a hand wand blender, blend for a minute to make rice cream. Season to taste.

Cream of Rice with Cardamom and Cranberries

• 3/4 cup short grain brown rice	• ½ cup oat groats
• 4 cups water	• ½ teaspoon salt
• ¼ teaspoon cardamom	• ½ cup dried cranberries

Use a 3-4 cup slow cooker. Combine all the dry ingredients , then add water, salt and cardamom. Cover and cook on low for 6-8 hours.

Stir in cranberries just before serving.

Millet Morning

• 1 cup millet	• 1 cup chopped dried fruit
• 1 ripe pear, peeled, chopped	• 1 teaspoon grated ginger
• 4-5 cups water	• ½ teaspoon salt

Rinse millet and toast in iron skillet for about 5 minutes. Stir constantly so it will not burn.

STOVETOP MILLET VERSION:

After toasting the millet, transfer it to a medium sized saucepan with water, fruit and ginger. Bring to a boil, then reduce heat to low, cover and simmer for 45 minutes until all liquid is absorbed. Top with chopped nuts as an option.

SLOW COOKER MILLET VERSION:

Transfer millet to a slow cooker, add remaining ingredients. Cover and cook for 6-8 hours on low.

Congee—Traditional Chinese Rice Porridge

• 1 cup short grain brown rice	• 1 cup yellow onion, minced
• 1 cup napa cabbage, fine	• 1 tablespoon minced ginger
• 1 clove garlic, minced	• 6 cups vegetable stock
• 1 tablespoon tamari	• Chopped scallion for garnish
• Chopped peanuts for garnish	

In slow cooker put rice, vegetables, garlic. Add stock and tamari, stir. Cover and cook for 6-8 hours on low. Garnish with scallions, peanuts and more tamari to taste.

Toasted Rice Cream

• 2 cups brown rice, rinsed	• 2 pinches of Celtic sea salt

We usually cook up about a cup of this rice at a time, leaving the rest for another day of the week.

Drain the rice. Toast it in a large cast iron skillet until dry and aroma becomes nutty. Cool, and then grind in a blender until consistency is coarse and sand like. In a small saucepan, for each cup of toasted rice, add 2½ cups water and a pinch of sea salt. Bring to a boil, and then simmer. Add more water during the cooking process if needed. Stir frequently, cook until creamy. Top with a dollop of coconut oil, raisins, nuts.

Store the rest of the toasted rice in an airtight container. It will keep for weeks.

David and Michelle's Morning Groats

• ¼ cup The Best Applesauce *	• ¾ cup sprouted groats
• 1 1" slice round pineapple	• 3 small pieces papaya or mango

Soak groats, (raw, organic, hulled buckwheat) in water for 15 minutes. After soaking, pour water from groats and rinse with water 2-3 times. After final rinse, put into mesh; covered mason jar and set upside down to drain. Keep upside down to sprout. Groats are ready when they have a ¼ inch shoot, in approximately 2-3 days. Be sure to rinse groats 2 times per day during this time.

When sprouts are ready, add to other ingredients in a blender for 3 minutes and serve. Add sliced banana or raisins if you like. Serves 3

Almond Cream

This delicious creamy topping is also from Joann's friends, Michelle and David. It is an excellent topping for most desserts or a bowl of fruit. It will keep for about. 2 -3 days.

• 1 cup whole almonds	• ½ cup water
• 1 teaspoon raw honey	• 1 teaspoon cinnamon

Soak the almonds for 12-24 hours. Peel soaked almonds. Blend the almonds with ½ cup of spring water until the mixture becomes thick (add more water if necessary). Add 1 teaspoon of honey and 1 teaspoon of cinnamon. Blend again, until very smooth. Refrigerate.

Barley and Kamut Breakfast Cereal

• ½ cup kamut	• ½ cup pearl barley
• ¼ cup oats	• 2 tablespoon sunflower seeds
• ½ cup mixed dried fruit	• ½ teaspoon cinnamon
• ½ teaspoon salt	• 4 cups water
• 1 teaspoon vanilla extract	• Pure maple syrup for topping

Combine the grains and sunflower seeds. Stir in dried fruit, cinnamon and salt. Then add water and vanilla. Mix. Cover and cook 6-8 hours on low over a flame tamer.

Overnight Oats

• 2 cups oats	• 8 ounces chopped pineapple
• 1 ½ cups rice milk or soy milk	• ½ teaspoon ground cardamom
• 1/8 teaspoon Celtic sea salt	• 1-2 ripe bananas
• ¼ cup ground flax seeds	• 1 ½ cups of water

Put all ingredients in a slow cooker, stir well. Cook on low for 6-8 hours

Muesli

• ½ cup cooked oat groats	• ¼ cup buckwheat groats
• ½ cup soy or rice milk	• Dash ground cinnamon
• 1 tablespoon raisins	• ½ apple, diced

Place oats, soy milk, cinnamon, and raisins in a bowl, stir to combine. Cover tightly with plastic wrap and refrigerate overnight. Just before serving, stir in apples.

Alternate: Blend ½ ripe banana and ¼ teaspoon vanilla extract until smooth. Add to muesli just before serving in place of cinnamon, raisins, and apple.

Or, top muesli with your favorite fruit: peaches, plums, apricots, pears, or berries of any kind. Toasted nuts are a great addition too.

Grain Bowls

(Scott could live on a "grain bowl" diet. Hunkering over a steaming bowl of whole grains and seasoned vegetables is probably his favorite way to eat. Use these as guidelines to create your own combinations with any foods you have available.)

Directions: Hold the bowl close. Let the steam hit your face. Use a spoon or chopsticks. Chew slow enough so your mouth savors the flavor. Say "ahh" and "mmm" once in a while.

Spring Grain Bowl
- Rice
- Asparagus and pea pods sautéed with capers
- Chickpeas
- Roasted garlic lemon sauce with chives

Summer Grain Bowl
- Quinoa
- Corn, zucchini, olive sauté
- Chopped scallions, Arugula, fresh basil or pesto

Fall Grain Bowl
- Millet
- Cauliflower sautéed with Thyme, sage, rosemary
- Ribbons of sea palm
- Chopped walnuts
- Quick & Tasty Tempeh with Mushroom Onion Sauce

Winter Grain Bowl

- Barley
- Roasted squash and root vegetables
- Sautéed kale
- Adzuki Beans
- Ginger Miso Tamari Sauce

Anytime Grain Bowl

- Brown Rice
- Sesame Tempeh
- Green Beans
- Spicy Thai Peanut Sauce

Ume Quinoa Grain Bowl

- Quinoa
- Avocado
- Cucumber
- Scallions
- Toasted pumpkin seeds
- Sprouts
- Ume vinegar and olive Oil

➤ BEAN & BEAN PRODUCTS

IMPORTANT: Please be sure to read the section called How To Make Beans Digestible. Learning to cook beans properly is a very important skill. Also read about Soybeans, under Food Controversies.

Savory Fava Beans with Capers, Garlic & Thyme

We have been preparing this dish with big Fava beans, and they are so meaty, you can really feel the protein in them. If you cannot find fava beans, you can use any larger legume. Cooking the beans from scratch will give you a chewier dish, but you can season any canned bean with these simple ingredients.

• 3 or 4 cups cooked fava beans	• ¼ cup olive oil
• 1 large clove garlic, minced	• ½ fresh lemon, juiced
• 1 teaspoon fresh sage, chopped	• ¼ teaspoon thyme, chopped
• ¼ cup flat leaf parsley, chopped	• 1 tablespoon salt-cured capers
• Celtic sea salt & ground pepper	• Chop the kombu and add in

Fava beans, or any larger bean work wonderfully for this recipe. Soak the beans 12 hours in spring or filtered water, change water a few times.

Rinse beans, cover with fresh water, add 3 inch piece of Kombu seaweed & cook, in a covered pot, over medium to low heat until tender (about 1-1 ½ hours, add water as needed). Or bring to pressure and cook for 3 minutes.

After beans have cooled, add olive oil, fresh squeezed lemon, chopped capers (the sea salt cured type), minced garlic, sage, thyme and parsley. Adjust salt and seasoning.

Kale, Chickpea & Pine Nuts

This dish is delicious served either hot or room temperature, but you can take it a step further and bake it in the oven over millet rice cakes in a 375 F oven for 20 minutes until the pine nuts and chickpeas get crisp.

• 2 tablespoon olive oil	• 1 bunch kale, thin ribbons
• 1/2 onion, chopped	• 2 cloves garlic, chopped
• 2 cups of cooked chickpeas	• 1 teaspoon fennel seeds
• Celtic sea salt	• 1/4 cup pine nuts

Heat 1 tablespoon olive oil in large sauté pan or skillet. Add onion and sauté for 5 minutes until golden. Add kale, 1/2 cup water and garlic, turn down heat to medium and steam sauté for 5-7 minutes. Next add chickpeas, pine nuts, fennel seeds and salt. Simmer for 15 minutes.

White Bean & Black Olive Spread

• 2 cups white/Northern beans	• 1 tablespoon tahini
• 1 whole head of garlic, roasted	• 1/2 fresh lime
• 10 black olives—kalamata	• 1/2 tablespoon basil or thyme
• 1/4 cup parsley	• 2-3 tablespoon water
• Celtic sea salt	

Roast garlic in a 425F oven by cutting off the top 1/8 " of the entire bulb. Drizzle a tiny amount of olive oil and cook in oven for 20 minutes. After garlic has cooled, add to food processor with tahini, olives, basil, parsley water and salt. Puree for 1 or 2 minutes, slowly adding oil. Use as spread, sauce or dip.

Quick Refried Beans

Having made your beans in advance, now its time to spice them up. The combinations are endless. Serve with rice, in a collard wrap or on top of a salad.

Sweet & Sour Tofu & Vegetables

• 1 medium onion, diced	• 3 tablespoon olive oil
• 1-2 cloves garlic, minced	• 2 cups shredded cabbage
• 1 cup snow pea pods	• 1 cup carrots, shredded
• ½ cup brown rice syrup	• 2 tablespoon tamari
• 2 tablespoon rice vinegar	• 8 oz tofu, ½ inch chunks

Heat oil in a wok or large sauté pan. Add garlic cabbage, carrots and stir fry for 5 minutes until soft. Add pea pods, tofu, brown rice syrup, tamari and rice vinegar and continue to cook on high heat for another 2–3 minutes. Serve over any grain.

Sautéed Corn & White Beans with Parsley

• 4-6 ears of fresh corn	• 1 small onion
• 3 tablespoon olive oil	• 2 cups cooked white beans
• 1/2 cup fresh parsley chopped	• Celtic sea salt
• Fresh ground pepper	

This is great when fresh corn is in season. However, frozen works well too. Cut the corn off the cobs (it will be easier to handle if you first cut the cob in half)

Heat the olive oil in a skillet over medium-high heat. Add onion and sauté until soft. Add corn and sauté for 8-10 minutes. Add cooked beans, parsley and salt and pepper, just long enough to heat beans through.

Raw Almond Hummus

• 1 cup raw almonds, soaked	• 1 clove garlic
• 1/2 teaspoon cumin seed	• 1 scallion, chopped
• 1/2 fresh squeezed lemon juice	• 1/2 teaspoon Celtic sea salt

Soak the almonds overnight (12-24 hours). Put all ingredients in a food processor, puree until texture is consistent. This won't be as smooth as chickpea hummus, but it is a nice change.

Chickpea Hummus

For roasted garlic hummus, gently heat 3 cloves of garlic in the oil until the garlic softens. Careful, don't brown it!

• 1/3 cup extra virgin olive oil	• 2 large cloves garlic, sliced thinly
• 2 teaspoon ground cumin	• 4 cups cooked garbanzo beans
• 3 tablespoon tahini	• 3 tablespoon fresh lemon juice
• 1 tablespoon miso	• 1/2 teaspoon Celtic sea salt

Put chickpeas, garlic, tahini, juice, salt and miso in the food processor. Mix for 20 seconds, add the oil slowly. Season to taste.

Tuscan Bean & Vegetable Salad

• 2 cups cooked cannellini beans	• 2 tablespoon flat leaf parsley, chopped
• 1 stalk celery, diced	• 1 tablespoon capers, minced
• 1/4 cup chopped black olives	• 1 head romaine lettuce, diced
• 1 tablespoon fresh basil leaves, minced	• 1/4 cup fresh lemon juice
• 6 tablespoon extra virgin olive oil	• 1 small red onion, diced
• Salt and pepper to taste	

Mix everything together.

Mexican Refried

• 2 cups beans, cooked	• 1 medium onion, diced
• 1 tablespoon olive oil	• ½ teaspoon cumin
• Juice of one lime	• 1 clove garlic, minced
• 1 inch ginger grated	

Start by sautéing up your onion until its soft. Add in cumin, chili if you like, coriander, garlic and ginger. Continue on low to medium heat for a couple minutes. Add the beans. Heat thoroughly.

Maple Refried Beans

A quick version of the timeless baked bean dish.

• 1 tablespoon olive oil	• 1 medium onion, diced
• 2 cups cooked navy beans	• 1/2 cup pure maple syrup
• 1 teaspoon dry mustard	• ½ teaspoon Celtic sea salt
• Freshly ground black pepper	

Heat the oil in a skillet, sauté the onion, cook until soft, about 5 minutes. Add other ingredients and cook for 5-8 minutes over medium low heat.

Curried Chickpeas

• 4 cups cooked chickpeas	• 2 tablespoon olive oil
• 1 large onion chopped fine	• 1 tablespoon fresh ginger
• 2 cloves garlic, minced	• 1 1/2 teaspoon curry powder
• 2 teaspoon ground cumin	• 4 cups kale, (or fresh spinach)
• 1 teaspoon salt	• 1 1/2 cups water

Heat oil in large skillet. Add onions and garlic. Cook until onions are golden, about 10 minutes. Add cumin and curry powder; stir constantly for 1 minute. Add the greens, water and salt. Reduce heat, cover and simmer until greens are cooked, approximately 7 minutes. Stir in chickpeas to heat through.

Cuban Black Beans

• 2 teaspoon olive oil	• 2 cloves garlic, minced
• ½ cup chopped onion	• 2 cups of cooked black beans
• 1 tablespoon tamari	• ½ cup chopped cilantro
• 1 teaspoon ground cumin	• Juice of a fresh lemon or lime
• Ground black pepper to taste	

Heat oil in saucepan over medium heat for one minute. Add garlic and onion, sauté for 5 minutes, stirring regularly. Add beans, tamari, cilantro, cumin, lemon and pepper. Reduce heat to low and cook for 10 minutes, or until ready to serve with hot sauce on the side.

Coconut Curry Tempeh

• 3 tablespoon coconut oil	• 16 ounces tempeh, ½" cubes
• ½ cup onions, thinly sliced	• 1 ½ teaspoons curry powder
• ½ teaspoon ground cumin	• 1/8 teaspoon dried red pepper
• 1 ½ teaspoon minced ginger	• 2 cloves garlic, minced
• 2 cups coconut milk	• 2 tablespoon cilantro, chopped

Heat the oil in a medium saucepan over medium heat. Add the onion and garlic. Cook for 5 minutes until soft. Add spices and cook for 1 minute. Add a bit of kuzu (a natural thickener) and cook for 1 minute. Stir in vegetable stock, slowly, then add, cilantro and coconut milk. Stir occasionally. Simmer for 20 minutes. You can store this in the refrigerator at this point. Add tempeh and simmer for another 20 minutes. You can also alternate tempeh with tofu.

Crispy Sesame Tempeh (or tofu)

• ½ cup sesame seeds	• 1 package tempeh
• 3 tablespoon olive oil	• 1 tablespoon tamari

Place the sesame seeds on a small plate. Dredge the tofu slices in 1 tablespoon olive oil, then the sesame seeds to coat on each side. In a large skillet, heat 2 tablespoons oil over med-high heat. Add the tempeh and cook until golden brown—about 3 minutes on each side. Just before turning, sprinkle with half tablespoon tamari on each side.

Quick & Tasty Tempeh (or tofu)

Once you make tempeh this way, you can add it to soups or use it with sauces and your choice of grain and vegetable.

• 1 tablespoon olive oil	• ½ tablespoon Tamari
• 3 cloves garlic, chopped	• 1 package Tempeh, ½" pieces
• Hot sauce (optional)	

Heat olive oil in skillet, add tempeh and sauté 3-4 minutes. Add garlic and tamari and continue to cook until the garlic softens.

Tempeh Quick Bake (or tofu)

• 1 package of tempeh	• 1-2 tablespoons of tamari

This is a quick way to bake tempeh whether you like the texture firm and drier or more stewed and soft. Either way, you can use the same seasonings and experiment with your favorite flavors. After its been baked, toss it into stir fry's, use in collard wraps or as a main dish.

One 8oz package of tempeh, cut into quarters and then quartered again. I like to slice it thinly so the flavors absorb easier but try whatever shape you like. You may even like to let it sit in a sauce for a while for a quick marinade.

Preheat oven to 350F. Place tempeh in a small baking dish, sprinkle with spices or toppings and tamari. Add about ½ inch of water, cover and bake for 35 minutes. For a drier texture, bake uncovered. For other flavors, add fennel seed, cumin and coriander, garlic, lemon juice, black pepper, or basil.

Tempeh Chimi-Churri

Marinated in authentic Argentinean spicy sauce. This recipe will pep up tempeh. It cooks great on the grill or baked in the oven. Lighter marinades work well with Tempeh as they absorb easier and send the flavor through the entire piece.

• ½ -1 cup parsley	• 8 garlic cloves, crushed
• ½ cup extra virgin olive oil	• ¼ cup apple cider vinegar
• ¼ teaspoon chili peppers	• 1 teaspoon dried oregano
• 1 teaspoon cumin	• ½ teaspoon Celtic Sea Salt
• Fresh ground pepper	• Bay Leaves
• ¼ cup lemon juice	• 1 packet of tempeh

Chop up parsley and cloves of garlic, mix into base of olive oil and vinegar. Add all other ingredients. Marinate the tempeh in the sauce for about 30 minutes. Cook in a skillet over medium-high heat for about 5 minutes each side. This sauce will keep in the refrigerator for at least a month. It works well with Tempeh, fish or tofu.

Tofu Scramble

You can add whatever you like, red pepper, pea pods, spices like cumin or fresh basil—use your imagination and whatever is available in your kitchen.

• ½ cup onion , minced	• ½ cup carrots ,diced
• ½ celery, diced	• ½ cup fresh parsley, minced
• 1 tub firm tofu, crumbled	• 1 teaspoon Celtic sea salt
• Fresh ground pepper	• Extra virgin olive oil
• ½ teaspoon turmeric	

Heat oil in shallow sauté pan or frying pan and add onions and carrots and celery. Cook until soft about 7 minutes. Add parsley and turmeric, salt and pepper and mix thoroughly. Add tofu and to stir fry for about 5 minutes.

Beans Fast Track Pressure Cooking

Use three cups of water to each cup of beans. Do not fill the pressure cooker more than half full, to prevent the pressure release valve from clogging. After you have measured everything out, seal up pressure cooker and bring up to pressure. Once your pressure has been reached, time the beans according to the list below. After the time is up, let the pressure come down naturally. Open the cooker and drain the beans.

- Large: fava, scarlet runners. Cook for 10 minutes under pressure, then allow pressure to come down .
- Medium Beans: chickpeas , pintos, black beans. Cook for 3 minutes under pressure then allow pressure to come down.
- Small beans: navy, or aduki. Cook for 2 minutes under pressure then allow pressure to come down.
- Test to assure their doneness, If for any reason, they need more cooking, easy, just simmer until ready with the lid on but not locked.

➤ Soups & Stews

Miso Quickie

• 8–10 oz boiled water	• 2 tablespoon chickpea miso
• 1 clove garlic, crushed	• Grated ginger juice

Let your water cool down a bit after boiling. Then in a cup or mug, dissolve misos. Then squeeze the fresh ginger into it.

To squeeze fresh ginger: the easy way to do it is to grate it and then just pick it up in your fingertips and squeeze into your recipe. About 1 tablespoon of grated ginger will yield about 1 teaspoon of juice.

Dashi:

Dashi is considered by some as the essence of Japanese cooking. It is a soup stock that is the most basic infusion of the sea prepared with the sea vegetable kombu and if you like, bonito flakes, a preserved fish fillet (skipjack) steamed, dried and shaved into flakes. It is a simple base for many dishes, the richness and depth of taste is incredible, offering the essence of the sea to any dish you prepare with this stock.

From dashi, you can make almost any soup or sauce. Plus you can make this stock in 10 minutes.

• ½ oz piece of kombu	• 1 quart of water
• 1 ounce of dried bonito flakes	

Heat the kombu and water slowly in medium saucepan. Just before boiling, take out the kombu so the foaming scum won't occur. Add bonito and turn off the heat. The bonito will sink to the bottom. Then strain through a fine sieve.

Miso Soup

The variations of this soup are endless. If you have miso and one or two vegetables in your refrigerator then you can make a deeply satisfying and nourishing soup.

• 4 inch wakame seaweed, rinsed	• 6–7 cups water
• 2 tablespoon miso	• 3-4 scallions, chopped

Any mix of vegetables will work, carrots and onions, cabbage and peas, daikon and scallion, kale, tofu and onion. It really can be left to your imagination. This combination will get you started.

Other variations: bring to a boil some wakame, onion, mushroom, and carrot in a heavy soup pot. Reduce heat and simmer, covered for 20 minutes or until your vegetables are tender. Take the miso and in a serrated suribachi (see Tools section) or bowl, dissolve with a couple cups of broth. Return the broth to the pot, making sure it does not boil. Simmer for 5 minutes, then garnish with fresh chopped scallions.

If you feel the need to add more miso for flavor, then dissolve another tablespoon to taste.

Another great variation for miso soup is to simmer bonito flakes with the wakame for 10 minutes, then strain before adding vegetables.

Stocks

Having your own soup stock will elevate the taste and quality of your food. Mostly you are controlling exactly what's going into your stock and you are using the same ingredients for other dishes, especially during your cleanse. You can make a large pot and freeze small containers to have ready to use. Freeze an ice cube tray's worth, then you'll have small flavor cubes to add to saute's and to cook your grains in. Just bag the cubes after they freeze to keep their flavor.

Vegetable Stock

A, clear stock, mild in flavor. Great way to use up any old vegetables or vegetable scraps. Avoid using cabbage, broccoli, cauliflower, collards. The flavors are too overpowering. Beets will turn your stock red.

• 4 quarts of water	• 1 onion
• 2 cloves garlic	• Leeks
• Carrots	• Celery
• Potatoes	• Greens
• Corn cobs	• Fennel
• Mushrooms	• Fresh parsley sprigs
• Celtic sea salt	

In a heavy stockpot bring your water and about 3 quarts of chopped vegetables and herbs to a boil. Reduce heat, skim if necessary and simmer for 1 ½ hours. Add water if you need to keep the vegetables covered. Pour soup through a strainer, pressing the vegetables as much as possible to get the most liquid out. Season to taste. Cool before refrigerating or freezing.

Sweet Potato, Chipotle Pepper & Kidney Bean Chili

• 1 tablespoon olive oil	• 1 medium sized onion, diced
• 1 tablespoon chili powder	• 1 large clove garlic, minced
• 1 ½ cups water	• 1 ½ lbs sweet potatoes, peeled
• 1 teaspoon ground coriander	• 2 cups kidney beans
• 1 teaspoon Celtic sea salt	• 1 teaspoon ground cumin
• 1 medium red bell pepper	• 2 medium tomatoes, diced
• 1 tablespoon canned chipotle peppers, or 1/4 teaspoon cayenne	

Feel free to use an assortment of sweet potatoes and yams with this recipe. Heat the oil in large skillet over med heat. Add the onion, bell pepper, garlic cover and cook until softened. Stir in the chili powder, other spices and cook for 30 seconds. Add the sweet potatoes and stir to coat with spices.

Transfer mixture to saucepan. Add the tomatoes, beans and water. Season with salt. Cover and cook for 45 minutes over medium high heat. When ready to serve, stir in chipolte peppers. Adjust seasonings to taste.

Spicy Thai Soup with Coconut Milk

This soup will be easy to prepare in under an hour and is so incredibly satisfying. Tackle it on a day when you are willing and able to spend your time there. First you make the soup base, then add the soup ingredients.

• 1 small onion, chopped	• 2" piece of ginger, sliced
• 5 cloves garlic, minced	• 2-3 fresh chili's, chopped
• 2 stalks lemon grass, 1" pieces	• 1 tablespoon ground coriander
• 1 teaspoon ground cumin seeds	• ½ teaspoon turmeric
• 2 teaspoon sweetener	• 2 tablespoon olive oil
• 5 cups water	• 1 can coconut milk (14 oz)
• ¼ cup fresh lime juice	• 1 teaspoon Celtic sea salt

Put the onion, ginger, garlic, chili, lemon grass, cumin, turmeric, coriander and brown rice syrup in a food processor. Puree into a paste. Heat the oil in a heavy soup pot over medium heat until hot, do not let it smoke. Add the paste and sauté, stirring often for about 8 minutes. Add the water, coconut milk, lime juice and salt and bring to a boil. Lower the heat and simmer for 30 minutes. Strain through a sieve and discard the solids. Return the broth to a clean pot and continue to simmer.

For the Soup:

• Cucumber, ½ cup, small pieces	• 1 cup mung bean sprouts
• 1 fresh jalapeno pepper, sliced	• ½ cup cilantro leaves, chopped
• ½ cup fresh mint, chopped	• 8 oz tofu, cut into ½ inch cubes
• 4 lime wedges	• 4 cups cooked quinoa

In individual bowls, add cucumber, sprouts, tofu, chilies and herbs.

Ladle the hot soup over cooked quinoa then mound the vegetable mixture in the middle and top with a lime wedge.

Creamy Squash Soup

This is a perfect soup for autumn and winter. It is warming, deeply nourishing, comforting and easy to prepare. There is also sweetness to this soup that is very satisfying.

• 2-3 lbs winter squash	• 1 tablespoon Olive oil
• 1 medium onion, chopped	• 2 stalks celery, chopped
• 1 apple, peeled and sliced	• 1 clove garlic, smashed
• 5-6 cups stock or water	• Salt
• Sage, 1 tablespoon chopped	• Thyme, 1 teaspoon fresh
• Scallion, thinly sliced	

Preheat oven to 450F. Halve the squash, place in a baking dish, cut side down and bake until tender, about 35-45 minutes.

In a large pot, heat the olive oil over medium heat and sauté the onion, celery, apple, garlic and a pinch of sea salt for 5 minutes. Add 1 cup water, sage, thyme and steam/sauté, covered, for 5-10 minutes or until very tender (add more water if it reduces to much).

After the squash is cooked and has slightly cooled. Remove the seeds and scoop the pulp from the skin and add to the vegetable mixture. Gradually stir in stock or water.

Blend until creamy; add more stock or water, if needed, to attain a creamy thick consistency (I like to use a hand held blender stick or you can transfer to a food processor). Adjust seasoning and serve, garnished with scallion slices.

Variations: add a can of coconut milk along with a teaspoon of curry and cumin powder.

Roasted Vegetable & White Bean Soup with Pesto

Use any vegetable you have on hand: squash, broccoli, asparagus, mushrooms.

• 3 tablespoon olive oil	• 2 large carrots, 1" pieces
• 1 large bulb fennel, 3/4 " pieces	• 3 ribs celery, 2" pieces
• 2 cups cauliflower, 1" pieces	• Celtic sea salt
• Pepper	• 4 cups vegetable broth or water
• 1 tablespoon rosemary & thyme	• 2 cups of cannellini beans

Heat over to 450º. In a large bowl put fennel, celery, carrots, and cauliflower, season with salt, pepper and olive oil. Spread on a large baking sheet, preferably with rims and roast tossing after 10 minutes and every 5 minutes thereafter until vegetables are brown and tender. Should take about 30 minutes. Let cool for 15 minutes and then either chop coarsely or leave whole.

In a large pot, put roasted vegetables, 4 cups vegetable broth or water, rosemary and beans. Bring to a boil, lower heat and simmer for 40 minutes. Before serving add a tablespoon of pesto to top.

Lentil & Escarole Soup

This soup really tastes better if you cook your lentils separately, then adding them to your greens. Try other greens like collards, kale, or mustard greens for some variety.

• 1 tablespoon olive oil	• 1 large onion, chopped
• 1 celery rib, chopped	• 1 large carrot, chopped
• 2 cloves garlic, minced	• 3/4 cup brown or green lentils
• 6 cups water	• 1 tablespoon tamari
• 1 teaspoon salt & pepper	• 4-5 large escarole leaves

Sauté onions in olive oil in a soup pot over medium heat. Add the celery, carrot and garlic. Cover and simmer on low until soft—about 8-10 minutes.

Roll the escarole leaves up and cut into thin ribbons. Add to vegetables with 4 cups water, tamari and cook on low for 45 minutes.

Cook the lentils. Add to soup. Season with Celtic sea salt and pepper.

Miso Shiitake Soup or Stew

This makes a great soup if you skip the quinoa step. Add other vegetables if you like.

• 4 tablespoon arame	• 7 cups water
• 4 teaspoon olive oil	• 1 medium onion, chopped
• 4 cloves garlic, sliced thinly	• 1 lb firm tofu
• 1 carrot, ½ moons, ¼" each	• 6 shiitake mushrooms
• 4" daikon radish, ¼" half moons	• 5-6 tablespoon red miso
• 2 cups bok choy (or cabbage)	• 2 teaspoon tamari
• 2 scallions thinly sliced	

Cut the tofu crosswise and into 1 inch cubes. Soak the arame in about ½ cup filtered water, set aside. Remove the stems from the shiitakes, and slice thinly, along with the bok choy and scallions.

In a 4-6 quart saucepan, cook onions in oil over medium–high heat until it begins to brown. Then add garlic and cook, stirring consistently for about 10 minutes.

Add tofu, shiitakes, carrots, daikon and remaining water about 6 cups; simmer for 40 minutes, covered until carrots are tender. Turn down heat.

Put miso in a small bowl with about 1 cup of stew broth, dissolve then return to stew.

Drain and rinse arame, add to stew. Add cabbage and tamari.

Serve with sliced scallions on top.

Miso Quinoa Stew

• ½ cup quinoa	• 2 cups water
• 1 piece kombu (1")	

Wash quinoa well, then put in small pan with kombu and 2 cups water. Bring to boil, reduce heat to low, cover and simmer for 35 minutes. Drain any excess water. Stir quinoa into stew after carrots are tender.

Veggie Jambalaya

Traditional jambalaya has a variety of meat, seafood or poultry added. Here you can use tempeh or seitan to replace part or all of the beans. Serve over hot, cooked rice.

• 1 tablespoon olive oil	• 2 cloves garlic, minced
• 2 ribs celery, ½ " pieces	• 3 or more cups water
• 3 cups cooked kidney beans	• 2 bay leaves, crushed
• 3/4 teaspoon dried thyme	• 1 teaspoon cayenne pepper
• 1 teaspoon dried oregano	• 1 teaspoon Celtic sea salt
• Chopped green onions	• Fresh parsley
• 8 oz Tempeh, ½ " pieces	

Heat oil in large skillet and sauté over medium heat onion, pepper, celery and garlic, about 5 minutes or until softened. In large saucepan, add sautéed vegetables to beans, water, and seasonings. Simmer for 25 minutes.

Just before serving, heat 1 tablespoon oil in small skillet and cook tempeh over medium high heat until browned. Add ground pepper for a spicy version. Mix into Jambalaya. Top with fresh parsley or chopped green onions. Add hot pepper for a spicier version.

Italian Vegetable Ragot

• 2 teaspoon olive oil	• 3 cloves garlic, minced
• 2 zucchini, ¼ " half moons	• 2 cups chopped kale
• 2 tablespoon kalamata olives	• 2 cups cooked white beans
• ¼ cup chopped fresh parsley	• 1 tablespoon salt-cured capers
• ¼ cup chopped fresh basil	• Salt and pepper

Remove spines from kale (save for juicing). In a 4 quart soup pot, sauté the garlic in olive oil for 3 minutes. Be careful not to burn it. Add zucchini and kale and continue to cook on medium heat for 4-5 minutes, then add beans, olives, capers and basil and enough water to make a soup. Bring to a slow boil, then lower heat to simmer for about 30-40 minutes, until the vegetables are cooked. Add pepper and top with fresh parsley.

Vegetarian Hot Pot

Using Dashi made with or without bonito would work well here, but it is not necessary.

• 5 cups filtered water	• 1 inch ginger, peeled and grated
• 2 cloves garlic, crushed	• 2 teaspoon olive oil
• 1 small onion, diced	• 2 cups shiitake mushrooms
• ¼ teaspoon crushed red pepper	• ½ teaspoon Celtic sea salt
• 1 small bok choy	• 10 oz tofu, ½ squares
• 1 cup grated carrots	• 4-6 teaspoon rice vinegar
• 2 teaspoon tamari	• 1 teaspoon toasted sesame oil
• 1/ 4 cup chopped scallions	

Combine broth, ginger, garlic in a large soup pot, bring to a simmer and cover over medium low heat for 15 minutes.

In a large skillet, heat oil. Add mushrooms and red pepper, cook, stirring frequently for 3-5 minutes. Add bok choy stems, and cook until tender, about 5 minutes.

Add mushroom mix to broth, and heat thoroughly for 3 minutes. Add bok choy greens, tofu and heat again 2 more minutes. Add carrots, vinegar to taste, tamari and sesame oil. Garnish with scallions.

Potato Leek Soup

Julia Child perfected this simple recipe, except she adds butter or whipping cream. Its delicious without and a snap to make.

• 3-4 cups potatoes, peeled	• 3 cups leeks, thinly sliced
• 64 oz water	• 1 tablespoon Celtic sea salt
• Black pepper to taste.	• 2-3 tablespoons parsley or chives

Cut the leeks lengthwise in half. Wash carefully to get out any dirt. Thinly slice into half moons (include the entire length of the leek). Simmer the vegetables, water and salt together for 40-50 minutes, partially covered. Mash the vegetables with a fork or pass through a sieve for a finer texture. Top with herbs before serving.

Fish Stew

This classic Italian fish soup has some interesting tastes thrown in. First it has cucumber that lightens the soup's flavor and mace, a spice that works well because of its sweetness. Mace is the thin lace-like covering over the shell of nutmeg, so its flavor is more delicate than nutmeg.

• 1 pound total of fresh white fish	• 1 teaspoon Celtic sea salt
• A small onion, sliced thinly	• ½ lb tomatoes, chopped
• ½ cucumber, chopped	• ½ cup parsley
• 2 oz olive oil	• ¼ pint of water
• Black pepper	• 1/8 teaspoon mace
• 2–3 bay leaves	• 3 cloves garlic

To make the broth, heat the olive oil in a pan, melt the sliced onion, add the cloves of garlic, chopped parsley, cucumber, the chopped tomatoes and bay leaves. Season with salt, pepper, and mace. Add the water and simmer for 20 minutes. If the broth is too thick, add more water. Cut the fish into thick slices removing the skin if possible. Put the fish in to the broth for about 5 minutes. Serve with more fresh chopped parsley on top.

Harvest Stew

• 2 leeks or 1 onion	• 2-3 carrots
• 1 small turnip	• 2 parsnips
• 1 cup winter squash	• 1 cup peas
• 2 potatoes	• 8" piece of burdock root
• 1 ½ cups celeriac or celery root	• 1 cup sliced mushrooms
• 2 tablespoons tamari	• 1 tablespoon of sage
• 2 tablespoons kuzu	• 1 tablespoon thyme & oregano

Cut the vegetables into 3/4-inch chunks. In a large soup pot, heat the olive oil and sauté your onions. Add the carrots, celery root, and burdock. Continue to sauté for a few more minutes. Add the rest of the vegetables, herbs, tamari and 3 cups of water. Bring to a boil, then reduce heat to simmer and cook for 25-30 minutes until vegetables are cooked. Dissolve kuzu in a ¼ cup of cold water. Add to stew to thicken. Adjust seasonings with salt and pepper.

Asian Seitan Soup with Cinnamon

Seitan is a "wheat meat" made by washing whole wheat grain until only the protein remains. You can find it prepared at most health food stores.

This soup has an interesting warming flavor with its combination of cinnamon, fennel and cilantro. You can easily substitute napa cabbage for the bok choy.

• 1 teaspoon sesame oil	• 3 cinnamon sticks
• 6 scallions, cut into ½" pieces	• 6 cloves garlic, minced
• 2 tablespoon ginger, minced	• 1 ½ teaspoon anise seeds
• 7 cups water	• 4 cups dashi or vegetable broth
• 1/3 cup tamari	• ¼ cup brown rice vinegar
• 8 ozs seitan, cut in thin strips	• 1 ½ pounds Napa cabbage
• ½ cup cilantro, chopped	

Heat the oil in a heavy soup pot over medium heat. When hot, add cinnamon, scallions, garlic, ginger and anise seeds stirring for 1 minute. Add the water, broth, tamari and vinegar and bring to boil over high heat. Lower the heat and add the seitan simmering over low heat for about 45 minutes.

Remove cinnamon sticks, add bok choy and simmer until stalks are tender about 5 minutes. Serve garnished with cilantro.

➤ VEGETABLE DISHES

Slow Cooker Artichokes

• 4 medium sized fresh artichokes	• Juice of 1 lemon
• 3 cups boiling water	• 3 cloves garlic, minced
• Celtic sea salt	

Mince garlic and mix with 1 teaspoon of salt. Cut off about an inch from top of the artichokes. Slice off the stem and trim pointy ends off the outer leaves. Spread the leaves out from the center a bit.

Spoon salt/ garlic mixture onto top of artichoke. Place the artichokes upright in 4 quart slow cooker.

Drizzle the lemon juice over the artichokes, then add the water to the cooker. Cover and cook on low for 6-8 hours, until tender. Serve either at room temperature or hot.

Asparagus with Lemon, Capers, and Onions

• 1 tablespoon olive oil	• 1 lb bunch of asparagus
• I medium onion, diced	• 1 tablespoon salt-cured capers
• Juice from ½ lemon	• Celtic sea salt and pepper

In a shallow pan, heat a few inches of water to boiling, add the asparagus and cook for 5-7 minutes. In another pan, heat olive oil and add onions, cook until translucent. Add capers, cook for a few more minutes until onions are tender. Add lemon juice and salt if needed. Toss asparagus with onion mixture.

Vegetable Burgers

Our friend Anthony worked out the recipe for these burgers. They are very easy to make.

• 3 cups sunflower seeds	• 2 carrots
• 1 teaspoon Celtic sea salt	• 1 clove garlic
• ½ teaspoon cumin	• 3 cups cooked brown rice, cooled or from refrigerator
• ¼–½ cup parsley	

In your food processor, combine all your ingredients until you have finely ground everything into a paste.

Form into patties and pan fry in olive oil for up to 10 minutes each side. These are great with the Chipotle pesto on top and fresh sauerkraut on top.

Jerusalem Artichoke, Peas and Shiitake Mushrooms

Jerusalem artichokes are full of iron and when cooked impart a wonderful nutty flavor. This recipe works well with peas or corn.

• 1 ½ cups Jerusalem artichokes	• 2 cups peas, frozen
• 5 shiitake mushrooms, slivered	• 1 medium onion, chopped
• 1 tablespoon olive oil	• 1 tablespoon tamari

In a large skillet, heat olive oil and then sauté onion until soft. Add shiitakes and tamari. Continue to cook for 4-6 minutes, just before mushrooms are cooked. Add peas and Jerusalem artichoke, some water and cook over medium-low heat until both are soft, approximately 5 more minutes. Add chopped parsley at the end and season with salt and pepper. Great with tofu, tempeh or fish.

Live Burritos (from Mikala)

First, make the Raw Cashew Sour Cream recipe: Put 2 cups of raw unsalted cashews in a jar with 4 cups of water, and let it soak over night.

In the morning strain and rinse the cashews well. Put the cashews in a blender with 1 cup of water and a dash of Celtic sea salt, and process very finely, adding water if necessary to get the consistency of sour cream. Place the cream in a glass bowl, and stir in the content of one capsule of any probiotic to start up the fermentation. Cover the bowl with cheesecloth held by a rubber band, and let it ferment a few hours in a warm place (on your counter, over a radiator, or in the sun). When covered with a tight lid, this cream keeps for many days in the refrigerator.

Put the following ingredients in a food processor and process until very fine:

• 2 teaspoon garlic, freshly peeled	• 2 teaspoon fresh ginger
• 1 teaspoon cumin	• 2 cups aduki bean sprouts
• 2 teaspoon Celtic sea salt	• 1 teaspoon fresh jalapenos pepper (or dried chili pepper)
• 2 tablespoon olive oil	

Mix in by hand:

• 3/4 cup fresh avocado

Lay this mixture over the large lettuce or cabbage leaves (steam the cabbage if it's too thick). Cover with the following:

• ¼ cup diced onion	• 3/4 cup freshly chopped cilantro
• 2 cups alfalfa or other sprouts	• 1 cup of cashew sour cream

Green Beans—quick and easy

• 1 lb fresh green beans	• 1-2 tablespoon olive oil
• Celtic sea salt	• Fresh lemon juice

Steam your green beans until they are bright green, and still crunchy. After they've cooled off, drizzle with olive oil and sea salt. Squeeze a bit of lemon if you like and you're done! Just like Grandma Rose used to make.

Queen Kinpira

The first time I tasted Kinpira, a carrot and burdock dish, I felt as if I were Japanese royalty, eating food that was extremely exotic, It's taste so perfectly even handed, both sweet and earthy, I wondered why I had never heard of it before. Kinpira turns out to be a traditional Japanese dish, simply meaning, sauté and simmer.

When strengthening and revitalizing burdock root is simmered with the sweetness of carrots, its rich, deep flavor is perfectly balanced. In our house we've added fresh grated ginger to this traditional dish.

• 3 burdock roots, each about 12 inches, cut into 2" matchsticks	• 2 large carrots, cut into 2" matchsticks
• 2 teaspoons dark sesame oil	• ¼ teaspoon Celtic sea salt
• 1 tablespoon tamari	• 1 tablespoon brown rice syrup
• 2 tablespoon water	• 1 tablespoon grated ginger

Heat sesame oil in heavy skillet over medium heat. Sauté burdock for several minutes. Lower heat then add water. Cover and cook for 10-15 minutes until burdock is tender. Add carrots, ginger, salt and sweetener, then sauté briefly. Cover and cook until tender, adding water to make sure the vegetables are not sticking to the pan. Season with tamari after removing from the heat.

Aduki Beans with Carrot, Kale and Hijiki

• 1 tablespoon olive oil	• ½ cup onion, chopped
• 2 cups aduki beans, cooked	• 1-2 cups carrot, matchsticks
• 1 -2 cups kale, thin strips	• 1 tablespoon dried hijiki
• 1 tablespoon Ginger, squeezed	• ½ teaspoon Celtic sea salt
• 2 tablespoon Tamari	• ½ cup water

Hydrate the hiziki for at least 15 minutes, then toss water. In a large sauté pan, heat the oil and add the onion. Cook for about 5 minutes until soft, add carrots and continue to cook for another 5 minutes. Then add kale and water to steam sauté the vegetables. Add aduki beans and ginger and stir frequently. Add tamari, salt and hijiki. Stir in well and adjust taste with tamari and black pepper.

Rutabagas Rustica

• 4 large rutabagas, peeled	• ¼ teaspoon Celtic sea salt
• Water	• 1 tablespoon olive oil
• Dash of nutmeg (optional)	• Pepper to taste

Cut rutabagas into chunks. Put them into a medium saucepan, add the salt and about 2" of water to cover. Cover saucepan, and bring to a boil over high heat. Turn heat down to medium and cook about 12-15 minutes, or until fork tender.

RUTABAGA OPTION 1:

Drain, reserving cooking liquid. Using a potato masher, coarsely mash rutabagas in the saucepan, adding cooking liquid as needed for moisture. Add olive oil Season to taste with salt and pepper. Transfer to a serving bowl, sprinkle with a dash of nutmeg, and garnish with a sprig of fresh sage or herb of your choice.

RUTABAGA OPTION 2:

Drain and leave in chunks, season with salt, pepper and olive oil.

Sweet Potato with Lime and Cilantro

• 3 sweet potatoes, 3/4" pieces	• 3 tablespoon olive oil
• 3/4 teaspoon Celtic sea salt	• ¼ teaspoon cayenne
• ½ teaspoon grated lime zest	• 1 tablespoon fresh lime juice
• ¼ cup freshly chopped cilantro	

Preheat oven to 425 degrees.

Toss sweet potatoes with 2 tablespoon olive oil and ¼ teaspoon salt. In shallow baking pan, arrange potatoes in a single layer. Roast for about 25 minutes, stirring half way through. Whisk together lime juice, cayenne, zest and remaining oil, then add potatoes, stirring gently. Toss with fresh cilantro.

Cooking greens

There are a lots of different ways of cooking greens like kale, collards, dandelions, and mustard greens. Weíve listed a few here. Once you find your favorite method, stick with it and youíll probably find youíre generally eating more greens on a regular basis. If you're using garlic with your recipe, add it after the greens have gone in the pan, so the garlic doesn't get bitter. Experiment with other flavors; you may like tamari instead of salt or replace the garlic with leeks.

Sautéed Greens with Garlic and Olive Oil

Leafy greens are one of those dishes you can eat every day. There is more calcium in a cup of cooked kale than in whole milk.

The recipes below apply to all greens: Collards, Kale, Dandelions, Mustard Greens. They also work for the oxalic acid greens, such as Swiss Chard and Spinach, but be careful with their usage. See the earlier section on oxalic acid.

Version 1: Joann's method

In a large skillet or suate pan, heat 1–2 tbsp olive oil over medium high heat. Add a bunch of freshly washed, greens, cut into bite size pieces or strips. Let the greens sizzle in the oil, turning them to let the oil coat all the greens and mix the water in. After they start to wilt, add a few cloves of chopped garlic, a teaspoon of Celtic sea salt and about a half cup more water, so as not to burn them. Cover and simmer until cooked.

Dress with fresh squeezed lemon and a touch more olive oil. Add raisins, currants, pine nuts or chopped almonds for variety. You can cook broccoli, cauliflower, green beans the same way.

VERSION 2: GARY'S METHOD (JOANN'S HUSBAND)

In a sauté pan or iron skillet, add ¼ inch water (add more water if needed), chopped pieces of kale or dandelions (any bitter greens) freshly washed, add finely chopped or crushed garlic (1-3 cloves), steam-sauté until tender. When greens are done (do not overcook) remove to a serving platter, drizzle with olive oil, sea salt or a dash of tamari to taste and the juice from ¼ to ½ lemon. Don't be surprised if you eat the entire dish.

VERSION 3: SCOTT'S "HURRY UP" METHOD

Push the whole bunch of leafy greens into water. Boil for 10 minutes. Drain, cut up the leaves and toss in olive oil, lemon and Celtic sea salt

Sesame Bok Choy

Bok choy is such a beautiful vegetable to eat on its own or with carrots. It's taste is mild so it's great if you want to add a wasabi sauce, grated ginger or hot peppers, to give it some punch. The benefits are incredible, especially because its one of the fat burning vegetables. This recipe has me eating it more regularly.

• 1 head bok choy, sliced thin	• 1 tablespoon olive oil
• 1 tablespoon sesame oil	• 2-3 teaspoon tamari
• 2 teaspoon sesame seeds	

Heat oil in a skillet, add bok choy and sauté on high heat, very quickly for a few minutes. As it wilts, add tamari and sesame seeds. Serve with hot sauces on side or just before serving. Serve immediately.

Sweet potatoes with Pineapple and Coconut

• 2 lbs sweet potatoes, peeled and cut into 2 " chunks	• ¼ cup unsweetened coconut
• ½ cup chopped pineapple	• ¼ teaspoon cinnamon
• 1 tablespoon maple syrup	

Mix together maple syrup, cinnamon and coconut. Stir in sweet potatoes, then spread in a baking pan. Bake at 350° for 40 minutes. Remove and stir in pineapple.

Green Coconut Potatoes

• Potatoes	• 1 can organic coconut milk
• Greens	• Salt or umeboshi vinegar

I am including this "recipe" to show how easy and fast a great tasting dish can be when you just make it up sometimes. It occurred one night a few months ago, after a long day of work and that state of mind where you open the refrigerator and think, "We have no food." I grabbed a bag of small organic potatoes, and put them into water on the stove (skins and all). While they were boiling, I opened up a can of organic coconut milk, added some greens (lettuce, broccoli, a couple of spring onions), seasoned it with some salt and umeboshi vinegar (one of my all time favorite flavors) and used a hand blender to make a green sauce. Once the potatoes were done, I quartered them (keeping the skins on) and poured over the sauce. Delicious.

Sea Palm: Weed of Darkness

• 1 cup dried Sea Palm seaweed	• Julienned jicama
• Salt or umebosh vinegar	• Dark sesame seed oil

Simmer the sea palm until al dente, about 15 minutes. Drain, rinse, and cut into 2" pieces. Make a simple dressing with umeboshi vinegar and the dark sesame oil. Toss in with the sea palm and jicama.

Indian Potato Croquettes

• 3–4 medium potatoes peeled, and cut into 2 " cubes	• 2 tablespoon-sunflower seeds ground in blender
• ½ teaspoon Celtic sea salt	• ¼ teaspoon turmeric
• ¼ teaspoon cumin	• 2 teaspoon canola or olive oil
• 1 teaspoon mustard seeds	• ¼ cup chopped parsley
• 2 tablespoon rice milk	

Cover potatoes in saucepan with water and boil. Cover and cook on medium until soft. Drain and transfer to large bowl and mash. Stir in parsley, salt and turmeric.

Heat 1 teaspoon oil in small skillet, add mustard seeds. When they start to pop, cover and add and cook for 15 seconds, stirring until golden brown. Add to potato mixture and mix well.

Divide the mixture into 12 balls and press into ½ in patty. Dip patty into rice milk and then coat with ground sunflowers. Heat 1 teaspoon oil in skillet and cook patties on medium heat until golden brown.

Maple Roasted Acorn Squash

• 2 acorn squash	• 3 tablespoon olive oil
• ½ teaspoon Celtic sea salt	• 2 tablespoon maple syrup
• 3 teaspoon minced ginger	• 4 tablespoon chopped pecans

Heat oven to 400º. Slice a thin piece off both ends of the squash, then cut the squash ion half. Scoop out the seeds. Oil the bottom of a baking dish that fit in the squash snugly. Smear the flesh with olive oil, then sprinkle salt, drizzle maple syrup and sprinkle with the ginger. Roast until nicely brown and tender, about 1 hour and 15 minutes. Add the pecans for the last 10 minutes. Don't undercook!

Roasted Salt & Pepper Squash

Cut squash in half, then length wise into slivered moon shapes, about ½ inch thin. Rub down with olive oil and broil on both sides until tender. Take a mix of Celtic sea salt and ground pepper and sprinkle generously before serving.

Sweet Potato Bake

• 2-3 sweet potatoes (about 1 ½ lbs), cut into 2 " cubes	• 1 tablespoon maple syrup
• 1 tablespoon tamari	• 1 tablespoon olive oil
• 2 tablespoon chopped pecans	• 2 tablespoon chopped walnuts

Preheat oven to 400º. Mix together maple syrup, tamari and olive oil. In a large bowl, toss potatoes with the liquid mixture. Put into shallow baking dish, covered and bake or 20 minutes. Remove top and bake for 15 more minutes until potatoes are cooked through. Add the chopped nuts for the last 5 minutes.

Mashed Potatoes, Turnips and Greens

• 3 medium russet potatoes,	• 3-4 medium turnips
• 1 sprig fresh thyme & fresh sage	• 4 teaspoon olive oil
• Celtic sea salt	• 2 large onions, sliced
• 4 cups greens: kale, broccoli rabe, mustard, or collards	

In a pot put potatoes, turnips and herbs, cover with water. Bring to a boil, then reduce to medium-high and cook uncovered until vegetables are tender 20 to 25 minutes. Drain, keeping the cooking liquid. Mash vegetables (discard the herbs) add 2 teaspoons oil and Celtic sea salt to taste. Add cooking water if needed. Set aside.

In another pan, sauté onions until golden and very tender, set aside. In a pot of water, cook greens until tender, then drain and add to onions. Serve potatoes topped with greens.

Onions Braised with Rosemary, Walnuts and Raisins.

This recipes works great with any onions, but try Vidalia or cippolini onion for variety.

• 3 cups sliced onions	• 2 tablespoon olive oil
• ½ cup water	• ½ cup golden raisins
• 1 teaspoon chopped rosemary	• ½ cup chopped walnuts

Heat oil in a large skillet. Add onion and cook until golden brown about 8 minutes. Add raisins, water and rosemary. Simmer for 20 minutes until onions are soft. Season with salt and pepper. Top with chopped walnuts just before serving.

Zucchini and Leek Sauté

• 1-2 tablespoon olive oil	• 1 large leek, cut into ½ " slices
• 1 teaspoon tamari	• 2-3 small zucchini, cut into ¼ inch half moons
• Celtic sea salt	

I always pick the smallest zucchini I can find, they're sweeter and more flavorful and combined with the sweetness of leeks it's a perfect combination of delicate flavor.

In a skillet heat the oil over medium-high heat. Add leeks and sauté for 4-5 minutes until soft and golden. Add zucchini and sea salt and continue on medium heat for another 4-5 minutes. When the zucchini is at your favorite consistency, add tamari and serve.

Capers and Onions and Parsley

Just imagine this dish with broiled tempeh, and herbed rice or inside a collard wrap.

• 1-2 tablespoon olive oil	• 3 onions, sliced thin
• ½ cup fresh parsley, chopped	• 3 tablespoon salt-cured capers, rinsed, drained and chopped
• Celtic sea salt	

Heat the olive oil in large skillet, add onions and sauté on medium heat until onions are translucent. Add capers and continue to sauté until the onions are syrupy brown. Remove from heat and add parsley and salt to taste.

Sautéed Corn, Beet Greens and Onion with Basil

• 4 ears corn	• 2 cups chopped beet greens
• 1 small onion, diced	• 2 tablespoon olive oil
• ¼ cup fresh basil, chopped	

This dish works well during fresh corn season, but frozen corn will do as well. Cut the kernels off from the corn cobs. In a skillet, heat your oil over medium to high heat, add onions and sauté until translucent, about 4 minutes. Add greens and corn and continue to cook on medium for another 5 minutes. Add basil and salt, before serving.

Collard Green Pesto

• 1 3/4 lb collard greens	• 7 large green olives
• 2 cloves garlic	• ½ cup water
• ½ teaspoon salt	• ½ cup olive oil

Cut out center ribs and stems from collard greens. Bring water to boil and stir in collards, then simmer about 15 minutes until tender. Save some cooking water and drain the leaves, gently pressing on them to extract excess water. Coarsely chop collards. In a food processor, blend olives, garlic, collards, water, salt and pulse until finely chopped. With motor running, slowly add oil.

Roasting Vegetables

This faster cooking method is easy to do with any vegetables and provides a richer taste without adding anything but good oil and salt to the vegetables. Afterwards you can choose to add the roasted vegetables to a salad or roll up or just eat them plain.

Here are some tips: cut all the vegetables to a uniform size. In a bowl toss them with olive oil. The oil will help them to become crisp on the outside and seal the flavors in. Transfer to a large baking sheet, big enough so the vegetables can lie in one layer. Roast at 425°, stirring every 10 minutes until they are fork tender.

Vegetables that are delicious roasted include leeks, asparagus, potatoes, beets, carrots, onions, squash. Herbs will enhance the flavor; add them when you are coating the vegetables with oil.

Roasted Root Vegetables

• 2 medium carrots, peeled	• 1 medium onion
• 1 medium sweet potato, peeled	• 8 oz mushrooms
• 2 medium parsnips	• 1 cup celery root, peeled
• 10 cloves garlic, peeled	• 3 tablespoon olive oil extra
• 1 tablespoon ume plum vinegar	• 2 teaspoon Celtic sea salt
• 1 tablespoon chopped rosemary or thyme	• ¼ cup chopped fresh parsley

Heat the oven to 425°. Cut all vegetables into 1" chunks. In a large bowl, toss all the vegetables with the olive oil, vinegar and salt, herbs. Spread the vegetables out (1 layer) in a baking dish and roast for about 50 minutes. Shake the pan up every 20 minutes. They will be done when tender and golden brown. Season with salt and pepper and top with fresh parsley.

Cabbage or Collard Green Roll Ups

Steam up a few whole collard greens or cabbage leaves and keep ready in fridge. I like to take out the heavy stem part of the collard and leave it for juicing. Don't prepare too many at a time, unless you plan to eat them up in a couple days. Add grains, beans, vegetables either raw, roasted or sautéed, nuts, sprouts, seeds, marinated arame, spicy thai peanut sauce, you name it, a collard green or cabbage leaf can handle it. And you will get that sandwich feeling, only better.

Italian Artichokes

• 4 medium sized fresh artichokes	• Juice of 1 lemon
• Celtic sea salt	• 1 tablespoon salt-cured capers
• 2 tablespoon olive oil	• Mince garlic
	• 1 teaspoon salt

Cut off about an inch from top of the artichokes. Slice off the stem and trim pointy ends off the outer leaves. Spread the leaves out from the center a bit. Rinse and drain.

Spoon capers and garlic on top of artichoke, stuffing into crevices as much as you can. Place the artichokes on a steamer upright in a large saucepan with about 2 inches of water in it. Squeeze lemon juice and drizzle oil over tops. Bring heat up to medium—high, but do not boil. Cover and simmer for 40 minutes until outer leaves are tender. Adjust seasonings if necessary.

Parslied Cauliflower

• 1 head cauliflower	• 2 tablespoons parsley, minced
• 2 tablespoons coconut oil	• 2 tablespoons olive oil
• salt and pepper to taste	

Steam the vegetables until soft. While still warm toss with oil, parsley,salt and pepper. Other ingredients you can add include red pepper flakes, lemon, chopped olives, pine nuts or capers. You can easily prepare broccoli, turnips, carrots, brussel sprouts, green beans, potatoes or squash in this same method.

Roasted Summer Squash

• 3 yellow squash, 6-8 inches	• 1 tablespoon fresh thyme
• 2 cloves garlic, slivers	• Red pepper flakes
• 1 ½ tablespoon pine nuts	• Salt and fresh ground pepper
• 1 tablespoon olive oil	

Preheat the oven to 400. Cut the squash in half, lengthwise. Scoop out the seeds and create a small cavity. Into each squash, put a couple slivers of garlic, a sprinkle of pine nuts, sprinkle of thyme and a sprinkle of red pepper flakes. Drizzle with olive oil and season with salt and pepper. Place the squash into a lightly oiled baking dish and cover. Bake for 25 minutes, remove foil and continue to cook on 300F for about 10 minutes until squash is soft.

Option: Top with Arame Tapenade after baking.

Sushi Salad

Sushi Salad is a favorite because it is so fast to make and you get all the flavors of sushi, avocado, cucumber, carrot, pickled ginger, sesame seeds and nori. You can of course, roll these ingredients, but the salad is a fun change.

• 2 cups cooked short brown rice	• 1 tablespoon brown rice vinegar
• 1 sheet Nori seaweed, strips	• 1 avocado peeled and cubed
• ½ cucumber, ½ "cubes	• 1 carrot, shaved with a peeler
• 1-2 tablespoon sesame seeds	• 3 scallions, sliced thinly
• 1 cup tofu, cut in ½" cubes	• 1 tablespoon olive oil
• Pickled ginger	• Wasabi, to taste

Cook your rice and transfer into a large bowl, wooden preferably. Drizzle brown rice vinegar over the rice as it's cooling. After it cools, add all the vegetables, seeds, tofu, olive oil, ginger and mix well. Top with nori strips and serve with wasabi on the side.

To make your brown rice a bit stickier than usual, you can adjust the water amount and cooking time. For 2 cups rice, use 4 cups water and if using a pressure cooker, cook for 5 more minutes. For variety, add slivered almonds and sprouts.

Corn on the Cob with Miso

Serve corn on the cob with chickpea or light miso as the spread and a squeeze of fresh lime juice. If you want a little kick, sprinkle with cayenne pepper or fresh ground black pepper

Marinated Arame

• ½ cup loosely packed arame	• 1 teaspoon tamari
• 1 teaspoon maple syrup	• 1 teaspoon ume vinegar

Rinse then soak the arame for 10 minutes, longer will dilute its flavor. Drain well and place in a bowl with tamari, vinegar and maple syrup. Let marinate for 15 minutes. Add to simple vegetable dishes or over rice. It will keep refrigerated for a few days. Try other seaweeds or a combination of them.

Cod with Rapini, Garlic and Olives

• 12 oz fresh Cod fillet	• 1 bunch of fresh rapini
• 4 cloves of garlic	• 1 tablespoon olive oil

Rapini, also known as broccoli rabe, is a leafy green vegetable commonly used in Chinese and Italian cuisine. Despite its name and appearance, it's actually not related to broccoli (most sources guess that it comes from the turnip family). While not common everywhere, try to find it, because it is very high in vitamins A, C, and K, as well as iron. If you can't locate rapini, use another leafy green.

Cut the rapini into bite size pieces. Heat the oil in a large skillet. Add the greens, the garlic and water. Steam the greens until almost cooked. Add the fish on top of the greens, a drizzle of olive oil, salt, pepper and olives. Check to make sure there is some liquid in the pan and add some if necessary. Cover and continue to steam for 8 minutes or longer if necessary.

Super Simple Carrots

• ½ tablespoon coconut oil	• ½ tablespoon olive oil
• 2 cups fresh carrots	• ½ teaspoon Celtic sea salt
• ½ cup water	

Cut the carrots into a consistent shape, such as chunks or spears. Heat the oil in a skillet before adding carrots. Sear for a minute or 2, then lower heat, add water and salt and cover until carrots are soft. Season with pepper.

This is the basic recipe for many vegetables. You can substitute carrots with nearly any other vegetable for a quick and tasty dish.

Wild Salmon with Miso Sesame Glaze

• 12 oz wild Salmon fillet	• 2 tablespoon miso
• 3 tablespoon pickle juice	• 1 tablespoon sesame seeds
• 1 tablespoon olive oil	• 1 clove garlic, minced
• ½ teaspoon ginger juice	

Natural pickle or sauerkraut brine is rich in friendly bacteria and a type of lactic acid that has shown to be a powerful immune enhancer. We use it in many dishes, not only for its health benefits, but for its great taste.

Blend together all ingredients except salmon. Cover salmon with sauce about an hour before cooking, refrigerate. In a skillet over medium heat add 1 tablespoon olive oil and put salmon in, skin side down. Cook slowly, with the lid on. There will be no need to turn the fish. Cooking time is approximately 10-12 minutes.

➤ SAUCES & DRESSINGS

Arame Tapenade

• 1 ounce of arame	• 1 clove garlic
• 2 tablespoon salt-cured capers	• 4 tablespoon kalamata olives
• ¼ cup red onion, chopped	• ¼ cup fresh basil
• 1 tablespoon olive oil	

Take an ounce of arame and pour boiling water over to cover; let sit for 10 minutes then drain well. In a food processor, first add garlic, then arame, capers, onion, kalamata olives and fresh basil. Add olive oil and chop to a paste.

Nut Butter with Lemon and Tamari

• 2 tablespoon nut butter	• 1 teaspoon tamari
• 1 tablespoon lemon juice	• 1 clove garlic, minced
• 1 tablespoon miso	• 4 tablespoon warm water
• Splash of hot sauce or cayenne	

Mix all together well in a bowl with a fork or with a hand blender

Basil Pesto

• 4 cups loosely packed basil	• 1 small clove garlic
• ¼ cup parsley	• Pepper & Celtic sea salt to taste
• 1 Tablespoon miso	• ½ cup toasted seeds (sunflower, walnuts, pine almonds)
• ¼ cup olive oil	

In a food processor blend basil, parsley, sunflower seeds, garlic, salt, and miso pulsing until finely chopped. Keep motor running and slowly add olive oil.

Black Cabbage Pesto

In Italy, they call lacinato kale, black cabbage. By either name, this is simply wonderful tasting and a great way to get kale into your diet. You can easily substitute collard greens.

• 1 3/4 lb lacinato kale	• ½ teaspoon salt
• 2 cloves garlic	• ½–½ cup olive oil
• 7 large green olives (¼ cup black kalamata work well too)	• ½ cup water (use the cooking water from the greens)

Cut out center ribs and stems from the kale. Bring a pot of water to boil and stir in greens, then simmer for about 15 minutes until tender. Save some cooking water and drain the leaves, gently pressing on them to extract excess water. Coarsely chop. In a food processor, blend olives, garlic, kale, water, and salt pulsing until finely chopped. With motor running, slowly add oil.

Cilantro Peanut Pesto

The parsley sweetens up the pesto; otherwise, the cilantro can be too bitter.

• 3 cups cilantro, loosely packed	• 1 cup parsley, loosely packed
• ½ cup peanuts, roasted	• 1 small clove garlic, peeled
• ½ cup olive oil	• ¼ teaspoon Celtic sea salt

In a food processor blend cilantro, parsley, peanuts, garlic, salt, pulsing until finely chopped. Keep motor running and slowly add olive oil.

Tahini Applesauce Spread

• ¼ cup tahini	• 3 apples, peeled, cored and diced. (pears work well too)
• 3 tablespoon light miso	

Blend all three until smooth with a hand blender. On toasted essene bread, this can easily become a new favorite.

Coconut Curry Sauce

Simmer vegetables or Tempeh, tofu or even fish in this sauce; its flavors work with a variety of foods. Its really great if you add an ingredient that you've prepared by quickly frying like crispy fish or Tempeh.

• 3 tablespoon olive oil	• 1 small onion
• 2 cloves garlic, peeled, chopped	• ½ teaspoon cumin
• 3/4 teaspoon Celtic sea salt	• 3 tablespoon curry powder
• 3 tablespoon kuzu	• 3 cups vegetable stock or water
• 2 cups coconut milk	• ½ cup cilantro, chopped

Heat the oil in a medium saucepan over medium heat. Add the onion and garlic. Cook for 5 minutes until soft. Add spices and cook for 1 minute. Add kuzu and cook for 1 minute. Stir in vegetable stock, slowly, then add cilantro and coconut milk. Stir occasionally. Simmer for 20 minutes. You can store this in the refrigerator at this point. Add vegetables or tofu and simmer for another 20 minutes.

Lemon Caper Sauce

• Juice of 2 lemons, ¼ cup	• ½ cup salt-cured capers
• 1 tablespoon tamari	• 1–2 cloves garlic, minced
• ½ cup olive oil	• 1 teaspoon prepared mustard
• 1/8 teaspoon salt	• 1/8 teaspoon ground pepper

In a small bowl, whisk together lemon juice, mustard and garlic. Slowly whisk in the olive oil until the mixture begins to emulsify. Stir in capers, black pepper and salt.

Raw Cashew Sour Cream (from Mikala)

• 2 cups cashews	• Salt
• 1 capsule probiotic	

Soak the 2 cups of raw unsalted cashews overnight in a jar with 4 cups water.

In the morning strain and rinse the cashews well. Put the cashews in a blender with 1 cup of water and a dash of Celtic sea salt, and process very finely, adding water if necessary to get the consistency of sour cream. Place the cream in a glass bowl, and stir in the content of one capsule of any probiotic (such as acidophilus) to start up the fermentation. Cover the bowl with cheesecloth held by a rubber band, and let it ferment a few hours in a warm place (on your counter, over a radiator, or in the sun; don't let it get over about 90 degrees). When covered with a tight lid, this cream keeps for many days in the refrigerator. Use with any recipe that would taste good with sour cream.

MISO SAUCES:

These are easy and as varied as you like. Miso and nut butters are a perfect combination and the variety is endless because you have at least 3 misos to choose from: light, medium or dark and 3 nut butters plus tahini and sunflower butter as well. Next you will need a liquid to thin it out. Choose from water, lemon, lime or orange juice, dashi or any soup stock. Then you can add garlic or ginger or both and for a bit more zip add hot sauce. Any type of chopped herb, parsley, basil, cilantro will do.

Here's a basic rule of thumb:

• 1 tablespoon of miso	• 1 tablespoon of nut butter
• 4 tablespoon of water or liquid	• 2 tablespoons of fresh herbs

Your wand blender will whip these sauces and dressings up in no time.

Spicy Thai Peanut Sauce

• 2 tablespoon olive oil	• ¼ cup scallions, finely chopped
• 1 clove garlic, finely chopped	• 1 tablespoon ginger root, grated
• 1 cup water	• ½ cup peanut butter
• ¼ cup tamari	• ¼ cup rice vinegar
• 3 tablespoon maple syrup	• Dash hot red pepper or cayenne

In a saucepan, heat oil over moderate heat until hot but not smoking. Cook scallions, garlic and ginger, stirring, until fragrant—about 1 minute. Stir in remaining ingredients and bring to a simmer, stirring constantly until mixture is smooth. Cool to room temperature. Add 1 cup of coconut milk before simmering for spicy coconut sauce.

Sesame Miso Maple Sauce

• 2 tablespoon sesame oil,	• 2 tablespoon olive oil
• 4 tablespoon tahini (or peanut)	• 4 tablespoon miso
• 5 tablespoon water	• 2 tablespoon maple syrup
• 1 teaspoon grated orange zest	

Mix this up in a covered jar to use on potatoes, salads, grains, or vegetables.

Ginger Miso Lime Sauce

• 3 tablespoon olive oil	• 3 tablespoon light miso
• ¼ cup water	• 1 clove crushed garlic or minced
• 1 tablespoon ginger, grated	• ¼ cup fresh lime juice
• 1 teaspoon maple syrup	• ½ teaspoon crushed red pepper

Dissolve miso in water, add all other ingredients and whisk until smooth.

Try this sauce on roasted vegetables like squash or pumpkin. You can add it to the vegetables while in the oven, but be sure to cover so the sauce will absorb into the food and not evaporate.

Classic Middle Eastern Tahini sauce

• ½ cup tahini	• 1-2 cloves garlic, minced
• 2 tablespoon fresh lemon juice	

In a small bowl, put tahini, garlic, lemon juice and sea salt, stirring constantly. Slowly add water to thin. This sauce can be used on falafel, grains, or even as a salad dressing.

Mushroom Onion Sauce

• 2 cups thinly sliced mushrooms	• 2 cups thinly sliced onions
• 2–3 tablespoon olive oil	• 1 ½ cups water
• 2 tablespoon tamari	• 1 ½ tablespoon kuzu
• ½ teaspoon sage	

Heat oil in skillet over high heat. Saute onions until they are golden brown. Add mushrooms and herbs, continue sautéing until they are soft and have lost most of their liquid. In a separate bowl, dissolve kuzu in water. Add to mushroom and onion mixture, stirring until thick. Remove from heat and add tamari. Use for any grain dishes.

Mango Orange Sauce

Delicious over other fruit or your morning breakfast cereal.

• ½ cup pure maple syrup	• 1/½ teaspoon orange zest
• ¼ cup water	• 1 tablespoon kuzu
• ½ cup fresh orange juice	• 1 tablespoon lemon juice, fresh
• 1 ripe mango, peeled, cubed	• ¼ teaspoon vanilla extract

In a small saucepan, simmer the maple syrup and orange zest for 3 minutes. Dissolve the kudzu in water. Add to the maple mixture and bring to a boil, stirring constantly with a wooden spoon. After the sauce thickens, remove from heat. Add the orange, lemon juice and vanilla. Strain through a fine sieve and let cool completely. Stir in the diced mango.

Walnut Miso Topping

• 1 cup walnuts	• 1 tablespoon water to thin
• ¼ cup red or barley miso	• 2-3 tablespoon brown rice syrup

Roast nuts in a skillet for about 5 minutes, then chop finely. Warm all ingredients on medium heat. Do not boil, it will ruin the miso. Simmer for 2-3 minutes until mixture thickens. Remove from heat and let cool before serving. Try it over cut up fruits, on essene bread or over grain dishes. Cashews, almonds or pecans will work equally well with this recipe.

Mango Relish

• 1 mango, peeled and diced	• 1 teaspoon maple syrup (optional)
• 3-5 scallions, sliced thinly	• 2 tablespoon cilantro or parsley
• Juice of one lime	• 1/8 teaspoon Celtic sea salt

Mix all ingredients together well in bowl, squeezing the lime last. Mix again and refrigerate for ½ hour.

Broiled Seitan with Broccoli & Mushroom Burdock Sauce

• 1 small onion, chopped	• 1 tbsp extra virgin olive oil
• ½ tbsp coconut oil	• 3 cups broccoli crowns
• 6 shitake or cremini mushrooms	• 1–6 " piece burdock root
• 3/4 cup water	• 2 tbsp tamari

Remove the stems and slice the mushrooms. Julienne the burdock root. Heat the oil in a large skillet, sauté onion until translucent over medium high heat. Add burdock root, mushrooms, broccoli, tamari and water. Continue to cook over medium heat until vegetables are cooked.

In a shallow baking sheet, line sliced seitan drizzled with olive oil. Broil until just crispy on both sides, about 4-5 minutes. Add to mushroom broccoli sauce.

Roasted Garlic Lemon Sauce

• 1 bulb garlic	• 2 tablespoons olive oil
• 1 teaspoon salt	• 1 teaspoon miso
• 2 tablespoons lemon juice	• 1 cup water

Peel away outer layers of garlic and slice off the tapered end. Drizzle with olive oil and put on baking sheet, cut side up. Roast garlic in 400F oven for about 30 minutes. Cool and remove from skins. Blend with the rest of the olive oil, lemon juice miso and salt and water until smooth.

Gomasio (sesame seeds and sea salt)

• 1 cup sesame seeds	• 1 teaspoon Celtic gray salt

Toast the seeds in a dry skillet until they just begin to color (careful, as they go from brown to *really* brown really fast). Use medium heat to start, and stir constantly with a wooden spoon. Pour them into your suribachi (described in the Tool section). While still hot, grind them with the wooden pestle, and then add the salt, and grind the two together into a nice course mixture. This will coat the salt with the oil from the seeds. Store in an airtight glass jar, to avoid oxidation.

Super Seed Gomasio

Here is a twist that pumps up the flavor, variety and nutrients. Toast all ingredients in the same manner, but separately.

• ¼ cup flax seeds, toasted	• ¼ cup sesame seeds, toasted
• 2 teaspoon Celtic sea salt	• ½ cup sea palm, toasted

After rinsing the flax seeds, toast lightly in an iron skillet or in the oven, Toast the sesame seeds the same way, Put both seeds in a herb grinder or suribachi with the sea salt and grind until the seeds have broken down. Add the toasted sea palm and grind that down. It should grind into a fine powder. Keep fresh in the refrigerator, but keep a small bowl nearby to top your grains, vegetables or salads. Again, store in an airtight glass jar.

Wasabi Sauce

• 3 tablespoon powdered wasabi	• 2 ½ tablespoon water
• 2 tablespoon tamari	• 8 tablespoon dashi

Blend. Yields 1 cup.

DRESSINGS

Dressings are just thinner versions of all the sauces we make. Just add olive oil, lemon juice, water or apple cider vinegar to any of the sauce recipes. They keep for a long time, so use a one quart mason jar, and make a few cups at a time.

➤ FERMENTED FOODS

Please do not skip fermented foods. I make this point because they are such a critical part of a cleansing and healing diet, and yet so many people don't eat them. Take the time to make your own large batch, or locate one of the very few (but growing) companies that make truly naturally fermented, non-pasteurized cultured vegetable foods.

Homemade cultured vegetables have become a recent phenomena, as more and more people realize that digestive problems are not there because of a lack of pharmaceutical drugs. Why use harsh prescription antibiotics and other medicine when the answer is right there in your kitchen? If you value a healthy digestive tract, you need cultured foods on a daily basis.

Get a Harsch vegetable fermenting ceramic pot. See the Tools section for its complete description. There is simply no easier way to create foods that contain friendly bacteria. The Harsch pot is one of those perfect tools that everyone who grasps the diet/disease, diet/symptom connection should own.

If you do not have a Harsch pot, just use a large (one or two gallon) glass container.

INTERESTING INFORMATION ON FERMENTATION:

The salting of the vegetables serves two major purposes. First, it causes an osmotic imbalance which results in the release of water and nutrients from the vegetable matter. The fluid expelled is an excellent growth medium for the microorganisms involved in the fermentation. It is rich in sugar and other growth factors. Second, the salt inhibits the growth of many spoilage organisms and pathogens that lie outside of normal human pH. It does not, obviously, inhibit the desired friendly bacteria. The actual salt concentration (brine strength) of these recipes is around 2 or 3 percent. While fermenting, it is important to keep oxygen out, as that would allow the growth of some spoilage organisms, particularly acid-loving molds and yeasts. This is why it's important to have all vegetable matter sitting under the brine.

Kimchi

• 9-10 pounds of Napa cabbage	• 2 onions
• 65 grams of Celtic Sea Salt, dissolved in 2 cups of pure water	• 20 tablespoons Korean chili powder
• 10-15 cloves garlic, crushed	• 1/2 cup dark sesame seed oil
• 25-40 spring onions, cut into 1 inch pieces	• 6-8 inches of fresh ginger root, peeled and grated
• 3 carrots & daikon radish, grated	• Optional: 1 cup chopped chives
• 5 Tablespoon of "kim chi sauce" (from an Oriental market)	• 10 tablespoonfuls of honey, agave syrup, or maple syrup

Shred the cabbage. Mix ingredients together. Place firmly in the bottom of your Harsch pot, or large glass jar. Place a clean rock on the top to keep everything under the resulting brine. Let ferment 10-14 days.

Mikala's Perfect Sauerkraut

• 20 pounds of organic cabbage	• 3 Tablespoon of fresh dill
• 3 Tablespoon of caraway seeds	• 120 grams salt (10 tablespoons)
• 70 juniper berries	• 8 capsules of friendly bacteria

Combine the ingredients (except for the cabbage) into a large bowl, and set aside (you can find juniper berries in specialty shops). From the 20 pounds of green cabbage, detach enough large outer leaves to form a 1/8" cover at the top of the crock; wash, dry and save them. Grate the rest of the cabbage.

Fill a Harsch Pickling Crock as follows: Place about 3 inches of grated cabbage at the bottom of the crock. Sprinkle in about 2 tablespoon of the seasoning. Add another 3 inches of grated cabbage. Pound down firmly to bring out the juice. Repeat this sequence, and be sure to finish off the seasoning before the last layer of cabbage. Cover the top with the large cabbage leaves.

Place the Harsch stoneware weights on top. Push down until the stones are covered with at least ½ inch of brine juice. Place the Harsch pot cover on, and fill up the water groove to prevent harmful entry of air and dust. Keep the crock at room temperature to encourage the fermentation process, and above the floor so that air can circulate. Let ferment undisturbed for 2 weeks. And be sure the water groove never goes empty.

Once done, transfer the sauerkraut into quart jars for ease of use. Make sure to tightly pack each jar, leaving ½" space before covering with lid. They will keep in the refrigerator up to several months.

Basic Pickles

• 6 pounds of small cucumbers	• 6 garlic cloves
• 4 dried or fresh sprigs dill weed	• 4 grape leaves (optional)
• 1 cup coarse Celtic gray sea salt	• 4 quarts water
• 10 peppercorns	• Harsch Pot, or gallon jar

Soak your cucumbers in very cold water for 10 minutes. Loosen any dirt, but no need to scrub them.

Pour some boiling or very hot water into your Harsch pot (or glass jar), swirl around, and empty it. This is a good last-minute way to sterilize your container.

Arrange the cucumbers, mixing in the grape leaf, garlic cloves and dill weed here and there.

Dissolve the sea salt in the water and pour this brine over the vegetables. Add the peppercorns.

Cover with the ceramic stones and push down, so that the brine covers the top of the cucumbers. Or, use a plate and a clean stone or brick if you're using a glass jar. Place the jar in a cool, dark place to ferment.

After 7-10 days, the cucumbers will be semi cured, and you can eat them like this. However, for the most zing, keep them going for three or four weeks.

If you're using a glass jar, skim the white yeast from the top once a week. With the Harsch pot, there won't be any, because of the air lock water gutter around the top rim.

Refrigerate the pickles to stop the fermentation process. Don't toss the liquid! It's where the most concentrated friendly flora are and it's a tasty pick me up.

Quick Pickles (see page 170)

Daikon & Red Cabbage Quick Pickle (see page 170)

166

SALADS

TIPS FOR GREAT SALADS:

Joann notes:

"Invest in a great knife; it is a tool that will undoubtedly bring you so much pleasure. I now almost exclusively use my Santoko knife, a Japanese chopper so light and sharp, it was worth every penny.

Get a salad spinner. It doesn't matter if it is fancy or cheap, as long as it spins your greens. I've used both and have had a five dollar version for four years now. When you have an extra moment, wash your greens, spin them, and store in bags in the fridge; they will be ready in a moment's notice.

Mix your flavors and textures. The stronger flavors of arugula and radicchio or dandelions add some punch to the milder, more delicate flavors of spinach and butterhead greens. Top with any a vegetable, grain, bean and a dressing.

Have your toppings ready. Get one of those divided Tupperware containers to keep shredded carrots, radish, sprouts, chickpeas, olives, cut up peppers, what ever you have and refill it regularly. Maybe you want a second one for all your roasted or raw nuts, seeds and fruits. I find it much easier to simply open one container.

The extras don't have to be raw vegetables. Think of grilled vegetables, roasted seeds and nuts, a scoop of leftover rice or quinoa. Roasted cubed potatoes work great as croutons. Pickled foods like sauerkraut or cut up dilled pickles add extra punch.

Make you favorite dressing in quantity. You can never go wrong with olive oil, lemon, salt and pepper.

Keep your dressings at work. At the very least, keep a bottle of olive oil at work, and maybe umeboshi vinegar and some Celtic sea salt. Then these items don't have to be packed up every day."

Asian Sesame Coleslaw

• ½ head cabbage, sliced thin.	• ½ cup shredded carrots
• ½ cup hijiki seaweed	• 1 tablespoon sesame seeds
• 1 teaspoon tamari	• 1-2 inch piece grated ginger
• 1 clove garlic, minced	• 2 tablespoon umembosi vinegar
• 2 tablespoon olive or flax oil.	• 1 complete scallion, sliced thin
• 3 tablespoon almond butter	• ¼ cup toasted sunflower seeds

Use any kind of cabbage for this dish. As always, you can substitute umeboshi vinegar with fresh lemon juice. Soak hijiki in water for 20 minutes, rinse and drain. Slice and shred your vegetables then toss with the nut butter, hijiki, garlic, ginger, sesame seeds, and dress with lemon juice, vinegar and oil. Add the nuts last so they don't get too soggy.

Fresh Fennel & Citrus Salad

This is when a really sharp knife can come in handy. Substitute 2 oranges for the 1 grapefruit for a change.

• 1 grapefruit, ½ sections	• 2 bulbs fresh fennel, sliced
• 1 tablespoon fresh lemon juice	• 1 tablespoon fresh lime juice
• 2 tablespoon olive oil	• Celtic sea salt
• Black Pepper, optional	• ½ teaspoon chopped sage

Chopped Arabic Salad

• 2 cucumbers	• 3 tablespoon olive oil
• 1 cup finely chopped red onion	• 1 cup purslane or spinach
• 1 cup finely chopped parsley	• ½ cup fresh mint, chopped
• 1 lemon	• 3/4 teaspoon Celtic sea salt

In one bowl, put all vegetables. In another smaller bowl put peeled and finely chopped lemon segments, keeping as much juice as possible. Add oil and salt and pepper to lemon, whisk together and dress vegetables.

Fast & Light Napa Cabbage Salad

My friend Susan made up this salad during a cleanse and ever since, Napa Cabbage has made its way as a regular salad in our house. This has a great blend of simple flavors.

• 1 head of Napa cabbage	• 2 navel oranges, peeled
• 1 ½ tablespoon tamari	• 3 tablespons olive oil
• ¼ cup tamari almonds	• Red onion (optional) ¼ cup

Shred the cabbage into thin strips, add sectioned oranges (or apples or plums) and tamari almonds . Dress with olive oil & tamari. If you are intolerant to mixing fruit and veggies, go with the citrus fruits for easier digestion. Pomegranate seeds are a perfect addition as well.

Carrot & Beet Salad

• 1 lb of carrots,	• 1-2 medium sized beets.
• ¼ cup currants or raisin	• 1 navel orange, peeled and cut
• 1/8 cup toasted pine nuts	• 3 tablespoon mint or basil
• 2 scallions, chopped	• 2 tablespoon fresh lime juice
• Olive oil	• Celtic sea salt

In a food processor, pulse carrots and beets until they are chopped pretty finely. Mix with all the other ingredients in a large bowl. As this sits, the vegetables will absorb the flavors more.

Jicama, Red Cabbage Salad with Sprouts and Lime

• 2 cups Jicama, julienned	• 4 cups red cabbage, shredded
• 1 cup mung sprouts	• Juice of 2 fresh limes
• Fresh ground pepper	• 3 tablespoon olive oil
• Celtic sea salt	

Jicama with Lime and Chili

This is a traditional Mexican way to eat jicama (hee'-kah-mah),a root vegetable with a nutty apple like flavor, high in vitamin C.

• 2 cups jicama, julienned	• 1 whole fresh squeezed lime
• Pinch of chili powder	• Salt to taste
• ¼ cup fresh cilantro, chopped	

Combine jicama, cilantro, oil, lime juice, salt and pepper. Gently toss to mix.

For a variation, try adding 2 navel oranges, peeled, quartered and sliced and 1
tablespoon olive oil and skip the cayenne pepper.

Mango & Avocado

• 1 firm mango, diced	• 1 avocado, peeled, chopped
• 2 tablespoon lemon juice	• 1 tablespoon lime juice
• 2 teaspoon minced green onion	• 1 jalapeño pepper, minced
• 1 tablespoon minced cilantro	• ¼ teaspoon Celtic sea salt

Stir all ingredients together . Serve at room temperature.

Sweet and Sour Cucumbers

• 3 cucumbers, sliced very thin	• 1 ½ teaspoon Celtic sea salt
• ½ cup lemon juice	• ¼ cup chopped fresh dill
• 2 tablespoon brown rice syrup	• Fresh ground pepper

Place cucumbers in colander and salt making sure all are coated. Let stand 15
minutes, shaking it up occasionally

Mix lemon juice, brown rice syrup dill and pepper in a separate bowl. Drain
cucumbers, pat dry and dress with mix. The longer you let them sit, the more
the flavors will blend.

Papa Joe's Celery & Olive Salad

• 2 bunches celery, including tops.	• ½ cup olive oil
• 1 Vidalia onion, 1" pieces	• 3 tablespoon flat leaf parsley
• 1 carrot shaved coarsely	• Juice of a whole lemon
• ¼ cup roasted red peppers	• 3/4 teaspoon Celtic sea salt
• Fresh ground pepper	• 1 ½ cups large green olives
• 1 ½ cups large black olives	

With celery dishes, try to always include the tops, which add flavor. Mix all ingredients together in a large bowl.

Quick Pickles

• 3 cups of any root vegetable	• 3 tablespoons of miso

An excellent use for root vegetables like kohlrabi, turnips and beets. Slice the vegetables into thin strips. Mix the miso with a little water and pour over vegetables. Let it sit, marinating for a few hours. Drain, reserving liquid (which you can use to create a salad dressing).

Daikon & Red Cabbage Quick Pickle

• 1 cup daikon, shredded	• 3 cups red cabbage, sliced thinly
• 1 teaspoon Celtic sea salt	• 1 tablespoon sesame seeds
• 2 tablespoon fresh lemon juice	• Juice of ½ orange
• 1 tablespoon orange zest	• 1 tablespoon olive oil

Mix daikon radish and cabbage well in a bowl with sea salt. Cover with a plate and weigh it down for a couple hours maximum. You'll see a good amount of liquid come from the mixture. Drain off liquid, add oil, citrus juice, sesame seeds. Season with salt and pepper to taste.

Guacamole

• 2 ripe avocados, ripe	• 2 tablespoon fresh lemon juice
• 2 cloves garlic, minced	• ½ teaspoon Celtic sea salt
• 1 tablespoon fresh cilantro	

Cut the avocados in half, remove pit and scoop out of its shell. In a bowl, drizzle lemon juice over the avocados and mash with a fork. Add the garlic, cilantro and if you'd like some ground pepper. Serve immediately or store with the pit to avoid discoloration of the avocado. For variety add ½ cup toasted pumpkin seeds that have been ground up in your food processor.

Pomegranate salad

• 1 medium sized pomegranate	• 2 medium ripe bananas
• 2 tablespoon fresh lime juice	• 1 tablespoon maple syrup or brown rice syrup
• ¼ teaspoon Celtic sea salt	

Cut the Pomegranate into quarters and soak in water for 5 minutes to help loosen the seeds. Twist each wedge to loosen the cells. Gently remove the seeds and arrange in a mound on a plate. Peel the bananas and slice on the diagonal – ¼ inch slices and arrange around the pomegranate cells. Sprinkle the lime juice and sweetener and salt and eat immediately.

This *kachamber* or little salad is a classic North Indian dish.

➤ QUICK ENERGY FOODS & DESSERTS

IMPORTANT: Please read the section on Sweeteners, in the earlier Pantry section.

Sweets are seductive, and can easily be overused. But in small amounts, they can be fine for even a cleansing program.

Fruit Smoothies and Sorbets

Very easy. Buy organic frozen fruit (or fresh fruit and ice). Add a few cups of water, add a banana for sweetness (or a bit of one of the sweeteners), and a pinch of salt to your blender. Slowly add fruit until it becomes thick. Spoon into nice glassware and serve.

The difference between a smoothie and sorbet is just in the thickness. You want a smoothie drinkable; you sorbet spoon-able. The problem is that a blender will stop blending once the ingredients become too thick. At that point, the best trick I have found is to use a paint brush. Purchase a cheap 1 or 2 inch wide paint brush, and carefully use it to help the blender keep blending. Just push the fruit mash down along the sides. Even if the spinning blades slightly touch the brush, the brush moves out of the way. After beating up a few wooden spoons, I have found this to be the perfect blending tool.

The Best Applesauce

• 8 apples	• 1 teaspoon raw honey
• ½ teaspoon cinnamon	• Juice of one orange

Peel, core, and slice the apples. Blend all ingredients for 3 minutes until smooth.

Baked Peaches and Blueberries with crispy, nutty topping

• 2 cups of blueberries	• 9 cups sliced peaches
• ½ cup brown rice syrup	• 2 tablespoon of lemon zest
• ½ cup chopped nuts	• ½ teaspoon cinnamon

Toss fruit with maple syrup, zest and spice. Place in baking dish, sprinkle with nuts and cinnamon, and bake for 35 minutes in 400F oven. Cover with foil if the nuts are burning. It's done when the fruit is soft. You can use other combinations of fruit, other sweeteners, and pecans, walnuts, or almonds.

Creamy Nutty Topping

Again this will work with any nuts you choose. Delicious on fresh fruit or a bowl of rice

• 3 tablespoon of maple syrup	• 1.5 tablespoons of walnut oil
• 1/12 teaspoon vanilla extract	• Pinch of Celtic sea salt
• ½ cup firm tofu	

Blend together in a blender for at least ½ minute until very smooth and creamy. Will store up to 5 days in refrigerator.

Infused Syrups

• ¼ cup maple syrup	• ¼ cup brown rice syrup
• ½ cup water	• 1 sprig of rosemary

Heat maple and brown rice syrup with water until it simmers. Add the infusing ingredient, lower the heat and cook for 7 minutes. Other flavors to try include thyme, ginger, vanilla bean or mint. Chill the syrup and drizzle lightly over any fruit you choose. You can also add this syrup to a smoothie, iced tea or fresh squeezed lemonade. Try these other syrup combinations:

• Melons with ginger & mint syrup	• Apricots with thyme syrup.
• Mixed berries & vanilla syrup	• Peaches, nectarines & rosemary
• Apples with cinnamon & anise	

Brown Rice Pudding

• 2 ½ cups cooked brown rice	• 1 ½ cups soy (unsweetened)
• ½ cup brown rice syrup	• 1 teaspoon vanilla extract
• ½ teaspoon ground cinnamon	• Pinch of Celtic sea salt
• ½ cup golden raisins	• ½ cup walnuts

Use unsweetened soy or almond milk. Combine all ingredients except nuts and raisins and cover, Bring up to boil, then simmer on low for 1 ½ hours. Stir after 45 minutes and add raisins then. Serve warm with chopped walnuts.

Date Walnut Balls

• 3/4 cup loosely packed dates	• ½ cup walnuts
• 1 teaspoon	• ¼ cup unsweetened coconut

Put all ingredients except coconut in a food processor and process until the nuts and fruit is finely chopped and starts to clump together. Spread coconut out on a baking sheet. Form balls with the nut & fruit mixture by rolling about a teaspoonful in your hands. Roll in coconut and store in the refrigerator.

Cranberry Grapefruit Compote

When winter hits and you're needing some fruit this is so satisfying.

• 1 cup fresh or frozen cranberries	• 1 ½ cups water
• 1 tbsp orange zest	• ½ cup fresh orange juice
• 3 large red grapefruit	• ¼ cup maple syrup
• fresh mint or sage	

Peel and section the grapefruit. Bring cranberries, water, orange zest and cinnamon stick to a boil in a saucepan over medium heat. Cook for about 3-5 minutes until the cranberries begin to pop. Remove from heat, transfer to a large bowl and refrigerate for approximately 2 hours.

Before serving, add grapefruit and all juice. Garnish with mint or sage.

➤ SNACKS AND CRUNCH

Sometimes you might just need a bit of something crunchy and seeing that you're eliminating crackers, and chips this is a good time to open your horizons.

Crunchy: Roasted nuts, sunflower and pumpkin seeds are perfect foods to toast on top of the stove or in the oven. Add nori or sea palm and toss with tamari. Add a dash of cumin for a spicier taste.

Roasted nuts. Put any kind of seed or nut into a skillet. Heat over a medium high flame for about 5 minutes, constantly stirring with a wooden spoon (careful so they don't scorch). Pull them off and while still piping hot, spray or sprinkle tamari over them.

Seaweed crunches: Sea Palm is one of the mildest, tastiest sea vegetables packed with nutritional punch. You can crisp in up in a 250° oven for 2-3 minutes and add to nuts and dried fruits to make your own trail mixes.

Toasted coconut.

Raw carrots & celery or cucumber soaked in mild salt water.

➤ DRINKS

Miso Hit the Spot

• 2 teaspoons light miso	• 1-2 teaspoons grated ginger
• 2 teaspoons chopped scallions	

Put all ingredients in a mug, fill with hot (not boiling) water and drink. Great before bed.

Hot Toddy

• 1 fresh squeezed lemon	• 1 teaspoon of sweetener
• Pinch of cayenne (optional)	• Boiling water

Joann's Broth

• 1 cup celery or fennel leaves	• 1 cup finely shredded carrots
• ½ cup shredded spinach	• 1 shredded parsley
• 1 quart water	• Pepper to taste
• 1 teaspoon Celtic Sea Salt	• Maple syrup or brown rice syrup

Use finely chopped celery or fennel leaves. Put all vegetables in the quart of water, cover and simmer for about 25 minutes, then add seasonings and little sweetener. Let cook for a bit more. Strain and serve.

Potassium Broth

Potassium is involved in nerve function, which is probably why this broth has a way of relaxing and soothing after a long day. It is very rich in potassium and can be used as the base for other soups. It's made from the "scrap pile" of vegetables, so it is deeply satisfying to make; you feel like you are really using all of the plant. The original idea for this came from Dr. Richard Schulze.

• 25% potato peelings	• 25% carrot & beet peelings
• 25% chopped onions	• 25 % celery and dark greens
• A few cloves of garlic	• Hot peppers to taste
• Enough water to cover	• Salt

Bring up to boil, then simmer for 20 minutes. Strain and season to taste.

The Water Cure Drink

While this is not a drink in the normal sense of the word, it is a powerful tool for those that suffer from digestion disorders. First taught by Dr. F. Batmanghelidj, M.D., in his book, *Your Body's Many Cries for Water*, it is a deceptively simple method for allowing the digestive tract—and the myriad of related symptoms— to heal. What follows is an adaptation taught to me by nutritionist Russell Mariani, MS, who has used it with great success in his private practice for the past seven years.

1. In the morning, put at least one quart of warm, pure water in a glass jar. Anything over 80° is fine.

2. Add a pinch of Celtic gray sea salt (up to 1/4 teaspoon per quart).

3. Sip slowly and try to drink it within the first hour or so in the morning. Don't gulp or drink more than four ounces at a time, to avoid bloating and to allow the body to assimilate the water and minerals.

It often takes a few days to get use to doing this, but you will actually start craving this much water in the morning, once your cells start rehydrating.

"Drugs never cure disease. They merely hush the voice of nature's protest, and pull down the danger signals she erects along the pathway of transgression.

"Any poison taken into the system has to be reckoned with later on even though it palliates present symptoms. Pain may disappear, but the patient is left in a worse condition, though unconscious of it at the time."

DR. DANIEL. H. KRESS, M.D.

PART THREE

A SAMPLE 28 DAYS OF
RECIPES AND CLEANSING TIPS

A Sample 28-Day Program

This last section lays out a sample 28-day cleansing program for you to follow. It is designed so that each day can be seen by placing the book flat on your kitchen counter. It can be used a basic guideline, with daily recipes and reminders. However, there is no need to follow it exactly; you can use any combination of recipes that you would like. It is simply meant as a guide.

Things to Remember

Water

Cleansing requires a large amount of water; it is the body's great solvent, critical for eliminating the waste products that get produced in vast quantities during a cleansing period. So be sure you drink the suggested amount of pure water each day. The basic rule of thumb: half your body weight in ounces (for example, a 100 pound person would drink 50 ounces each day). We suggest getting a special rehydration jug, that you fill up each day. This is water you will drink aside from any tea, juice, or other liquids that you drink each day.

If you are suffering from digestion disorders, read the earlier section on the Water Cure, and add it to your daily regimen.

Juicing

Don't forget to drink at least 12 ounces of fresh vegetable juice each day. It is there on each day's program, already checked off.

7 Physical Transformers

On the lower left corner of each page, you will see the list of 7 PTs. Look ahead and try to check off at least one PT for each day. Some of them will be easy to do, such as dry brushing or alkaline baths; others, like the colon therapy and sauna rounds, are best scheduled in advance. That way, you stay committed to doing them.

SUPPLEMENTS AND SUPERFOODS

If you can budget for superfood supplements, do. They will increase your results, and give you more leeway with a non-perfect diet. The main ones are listed on each day's page.

CHEWING

When people call me, saying that they are not getting the results they want, one of the first things I tell them to do is this: **for the next week, don't swallow each bite until you feel your mouth release saliva.** Oftentimes, this single action and focus is the only thing they need to do to start seeing results. If we swallow our food, week after week after week, without surrounding each bite with saliva, we are not getting our body's natural enzymes. Slow down. Start to pay attention to chewing.

FOOD COMBINING

Four basic rules:

1. Don't mix sweeteners with oil (especially if you have skin problems)
2. Don't mix sweeteners with protein (especially if you have digestive problems)
3. If digestion is an issue, separate proteins from carbohydrates
4. Eat fruit alone: nothing after for 60 minutes, nothing before for 3 hours

DON'T GO HUNGRY

This is not a starvation program. It's a cleansing one. If you get hungry, you're probably not eating enough, or you are not drinking enough between meals. You are changing the fuel that your body is used to. Keep it calmed down by eating enough, drinking enough (both water and teas), and snacking enough. As long as it is cleansing food, and you are chewing thoroughly, eat as much as you want.

ANIMAL PROTEIN

If you are extremely physically active—you jog, or work out in a gym, etc.— and feel the need for animal food, add an occassional fresh organic egg with meals. Use the fish recipes. Remember: don't think volume, think energetics.

Add small amounts to broths and stews. Choose only the purest sources you can find. And NO MILK PRODUCTS. Period.

STOP USING TOXIC PERSONAL CARE PRODUCTS

It is nothing short of insanity what many people put on their skin or use to wash their clothes, or scent their bodies and homes, and make no association with skin, digestive, hormonal, or nervous system disorders. Hugging some-one often leaves me with the scent of toxic perfumes and hair spray on my clothes for hours and even the next day.

If you are trying to get healthy, you need to stop using most scents, soaps, shampoos and conditioners. You also need to stop using fabric softeners, most detergents, and most house surface cleaners. They are making yourself and your children and your animals sick. Fortunately, it is very easy to replace them with nontoxic products. Check your local health food store. Look for ones that have fewer ingredients and are scented with essential oils, or not scented at all.

DETOXIFICATION AND ENERGY LEVELS

If you clean out a pond and creek from years of debris, you will stir up that debris in the process. Initially, it can look like you are making matters worse, but eventually, the water is clearer than it was before.

Same goes with internal debris cleansing. Don't be alarmed if you go through a detoxification period. Most everyone does (we certainly do), and it lasts anywhere from 1 to 10 days.

Be kind to yourself if your energy and mental levels are not the same as always. Plan on napping more, or reading, or sitting quietly. It is part of what healing looks like.

GARLIC INFUSION AND OTHER MINI CLEANSES

One of my favorite things during a cleanse is to do small, focused mini cleanses. Here are some of my favorites:

1. Garlic Infusion. Find a time when you aren't going to be very social. Then for 3 to 5 days in a row, eat 5-15 cloves of raw garlic during each day. While you can crush them and add them to soup or dressings, I like to simply use my hand food chopper, and dice them up (2 or 3 at a time) into small 1/8" pieces. I then swish and swallow some water (to whet the mouth); I then put a small teaspoon of the chopped garlic in my mouth, and down it with a large glass of water. After awhile, you can get quite skilled at this, and be able to swallow quite a bit of garlic directly into the stomach.

This infuses the entire body with the anti-parasitic, anti-bacterial, and anti-viral and fungal properties of raw garlic. I believe that this single action is the main reason why I have not gotten a cold or flu in over 4 years. Very, very powerful.

2. Superfood Week. During one week, consume a large amount of encapsulated superfoods. I usually use do a variety of dried wild bluegreen algae, dried kelp, enzymes, friendly bacteria, and green drinks. I will do 2 or more shots of fresh wheatgrass each morning. Anything to increase the amount of chlorophyll going into my bloodstream for that week.

3. Colon Care. Although it is already strongly recommended during the cleanse, I like to focus on extra colon care for a week or so. I will schedule a couple of colonics during that time; I'll roll around and do reverse sit-ups on a physioball (those 24-inch diameter exercise balls) while watching TV at night (Sam Iannetta, owner of FunctionalFitnessUSA.com, says that this is one of the surest ways of alleviating constipation); I will mix small amounts of colon cleanser in water twice a day. Anything that helps strengthen and support the digestive system.

4. Intense Sauna Week. I will often do this one in the middle of the winter, even if I'm not doing any other kind of cleansing. Every night for 7-10 days, I will really sweat it out in a sauna. I try to stay in 60-120 minutes, taking breaks when I need to. I'll read, listen to audiobooks, or invite friends to join me.

5. Anti-Parasite program. It only takes one friend, telling you about the 12 inch worm that came out in their morning stool after a parasite-clearing program, to convince you to adding this to your mini cleanses. It is beyond the scope of this book to describe the different anti-parasite programs, but Dr. Nasha Winters from NamasteHealthCenter.com gets photograph-proof results with her clients by simply having them eat a handful of pumpkin seeds each day for 14 days. Start there, and visit HowHealthWorks.com for other ideas.

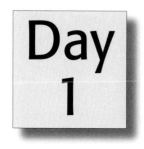

"My brother had ulcerated colitis. During and after this cleanse, his symptoms lessened dramatically and he was able to get off all medication. Thank you for this work."

LAUREN GENNETT

Check your pantry and refrigerator for:

• Oat groats	• Carrots, celery, cucumbers
• Brown Rice	• Jicama, sweet potato
	• Raisins
• Hummus	• Avocado
• Kidney Beans	• Lemon
	• Salad greens
• Dressing	• Walnuts
• Maple syrup	• Cumin Cinnamon Cilantro
• Ground coriander	• Chipotle peppers

7 Physical Transformers

☒ Rehydrate (EVERY DAY. Half your body weight in ounces of water)

Do at least one of the following each day:

☐ Skin Brushing

☐ Colon Cleanse

☐ Sauna Rounds

☐ Alkalinizing Bath

☐ Cleansing Bodywork

☐ Cardiovascular Sweat

Supplements & Superfoods

☒ 12–32 ounces of fresh vegetable juice. Every day.

☐ Probiotics (Acidophilus, etc)

☐ Green Drink

☐ Algae (freshwater or ocean)

☐ Enzymes

☐ Garlic clove or Allimax

☐ Colon cleansing products

BREAKFAST
Overnight Oat Groats with cinnamon, walnuts and raisins......... page 111

LUNCH
Hummus.. page 121
Guacamole, cut up raw vegetables .... page 171
Salad Greens

DINNER
Sweet Potato Chipotle Chili... page 128
Rice .... page 103
Salad or green vegetable
Tea

Notes & Journal: Day 1 of 28

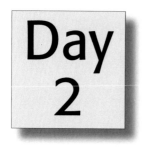

When diet is wrong, medicine is of no use. When diet is correct, medicine is of no need.

ANCIENT AYURVEDIC PROVERB

Check your pantry and refrigerator for:

• Essene bread	• Kale
	• Apple & assorted fresh fruit
	• Lettuce greens or sprouts
• Miso	• Winter squash
• Nut butter or tahini	• Celery
• Sunflower seeds	• Sage
• Coconut oil	• Collard greens
• Thyme	• Chickpeas
• Curry powder	• Scallions

7 Physical Transformers

☒ Rehydrate (EVERY DAY. Half your body weight in ounces of water)

Do at least one of the following each day:

☐ Skin Brushing

☐ Colon Cleanse

☐ Sauna Rounds

☐ Alkalinizing Bath

☐ Cleansing Bodywork

☐ Cardiovascular Sweat

Supplements & Superfoods

☒ 12–32 ounces of fresh vegetable juice. Every day.

☐ Probiotics (Acidophilus, etc)

☐ Green Drink

☐ Algae (freshwater or ocean)

☐ Enzymes

☐ Garlic clove or Allimax

☐ Colon cleansing products

BREAKFAST

Toasted Essene bread

Spread on coconut butter/oil, miso, nut spread and fresh fruit

LUNCH

Collard Green Roll ups .... page 150

Stuffed with rice, left over chili, lettuce, sunflower seeds

DINNER

Squash soup.. page 130

Curried chickpeas .... page 122

Fresh green salad with Roasted Garlic Lemon Dressing.............. page 161
(remember: dressings are simply sauces thinned out)

Tea

Notes & Journal: Day 2 of 28

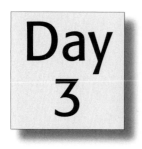

Day 3

Check your pantry and refrigerator for:

• Tempeh	• Assorted fresh fruit, oranges
• Rice	• Almonds
• Essene bread	• Red onion
• Sauerkraut	• Green beans
• Rice vinegar	• Napa Cabbage
• Peanut butter	• Cayenne or hot pepper sauce

7 Physical Transformers

☒ Rehydrate (EVERY DAY. Half your body weight in ounces of water)

Do at least one of the following each day:

☐ Skin Brushing

☐ Colon Cleanse

☐ Sauna Rounds

☐ Alkalinizing Bath

☐ Cleansing Bodywork

☐ Cardiovascular Sweat

Supplements & Superfoods

☒ 12–32 ounces of fresh vegetable juice. Every day.

☐ Probiotics (Acidophilus, etc)

☐ Green Drink

☐ Algae (freshwater or ocean)

☐ Enzymes

☐ Garlic clove or Allimax

☐ Colon cleansing products

Breakfast
Fresh fruit or Essene Bread

Lunch
Squash Soup (left over from yesterday) .... page 130

Fast and Light Napa Salad .... page 168

Dinner
Anytime Grain Bowl .... page 117

Sauerkraut .... page 163

Tea

Notes & Journal: Day 3 of 28

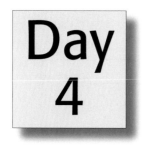

"It is nothing short of a miracle that the modern methods of instruction have not entirely strangled the holy curiosity of inquiry."

ALBERT EINSTEIN

Check your pantry and refrigerator for:

• Millet	• Carrot, potatoes, kale, scallions
• Brown rice	• Parsley and salad greens
	• Pears and lemons
• Fava beans	• Apricots or other dried fruit
• Capers	• Cilantro
• Miso Soup	• Sage, thyme and mustard seeds
• Rice milk	• Peanuts
• Tempeh	• Sunflower and sesame seeds

7 Physical Transformers

[X] Rehydrate (EVERY DAY. Half your body weight in ounces of water)

Do at least one of the following each day:

[ ] Skin Brushing

[ ] Colon Cleanse

[ ] Sauna Rounds

[ ] Alkalinizing Bath

[ ] Cleansing Bodywork

[ ] Cardiovascular Sweat

Supplements & Superfoods

[X] 12–32 ounces of fresh vegetable juice. Every day.

[ ] Probiotics (Acidophilus, etc)

[ ] Green Drink

[ ] Algae (freshwater or ocean)

[ ] Enzymes

[ ] Garlic clove or Allimax

[ ] Colon cleansing products

Breakfast

Remember: not all breakfasts need to be sweet; try a savory one.

Lunch

Dinner

Tea

Notes & Journal: Day 4 of 28

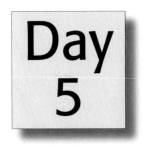

" I no longer suffer from acid reflux as I did before I started this detoxification program. Thank you for this."

MARIE ROY

Check your pantry and refrigerator for:

• Oat groats	• Carrot
• Rice	• Cauliflower
• Chickpeas	• Leeks
• Lime	• Shiitake mushrooms
• Arame	• Daikon radish
• Bok choy	• Scallion
• Tofu	

7 Physical Transformers

☒ Rehydrate (EVERY DAY. Half your body weight in ounces of water)

Do at least one of the following each day:

☐ Skin Brushing
☐ Colon Cleanse
☐ Sauna Rounds
☐ Alkalinizing Bath
☐ Cleansing Bodywork
☐ Cardiovascular Sweat

Supplements & Superfoods

☒ 12–32 ounces of fresh vegetable juice. Every day.

☐ Probiotics (Acidophilus, etc)
☐ Green Drink
☐ Algae (freshwater or ocean)
☐ Enzymes
☐ Garlic clove or Allimax
☐ Colon cleansing products

Breakfast
Oat Cream with sweet or savory topping .... page 111
Gomasio (optional) .... page 161

Lunch
Spring Grain Bowl .... page 116

Dinner
Miso Shiitake Soup .... page 132
Green Salad with any dressing
Tea

Notes & Journal: Day 5 of 28

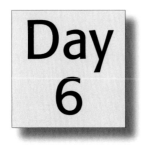

"Habit is habit and not to be flung out the window by anyone, but coaxed downstairs a step at a time.

MARK TWAIN

Check your pantry and refrigerator for:

• Essene bread	• Fresh tomato, celery, lemons
• Rice	• Mint
• Quinoa	• Escarole, parsley
• Miso Soup	• Curry powder
• Tofu	
• Lentils	• Cashews

7 Physical Transformers

☒ Rehydrate (EVERY DAY. Half your body weight in ounces of water)

Do at least one of the following each day:

☐ Skin Brushing

☐ Colon Cleanse

☐ Sauna Rounds

☐ Alkalinizing Bath

☐ Cleansing Bodywork

☐ Cardiovascular Sweat

Supplements & Superfoods

☒ 12–32 ounces of fresh vegetable juice. Every day.

☐ Probiotics (Acidophilus, etc)

☐ Green Drink

☐ Algae (freshwater or ocean)

☐ Enzymes

☐ Garlic clove or Allimax

☐ Colon cleansing products

BREAKFAST

Toasted Essene bread

LUNCH

DINNER

Tea

Notes & Journal: Day 6 of 28

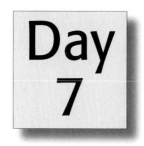

Day 7

"You don't have to do cleansing perfectly. Far from it. You only need to pay attention to what you eat each day. Constant incremental improvement: that's the key."

SCOTT OHLGREN

Check your pantry and refrigerator for:

• Rice with favorite toppings	• Carrots, Fennel
• Grapefruit	• Lime , Kale
	• Acorn squash
• Pecans	• Sage
• Aduki beans	• Maple syrup
• Hijiki	

7 Physical Transformers

☒ Rehydrate (EVERY DAY. Half your body weight in ounces of water)

Do at least one of the following each day:

☐ Skin Brushing

☐ Colon Cleanse

☐ Sauna Rounds

☐ Alkalinizing Bath

☐ Cleansing Bodywork

☐ Cardiovascular Sweat

Supplements & Superfoods

☒ 12–32 ounces of fresh vegetable juice. Every day.

☐ Probiotics (Acidophilus, etc)

☐ Green Drink

☐ Algae (freshwater or ocean)

☐ Enzymes

☐ Garlic clove or Allimax

☐ Colon cleansing products

BREAKFAST

LUNCH

DINNER
Tea

Notes & Journal: Day 7 of 28

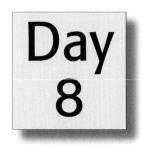

Day 8

"The greatest part of all chronic disease is created by the suppression of acute disease by drug poisoning."

Dr. Henry Lindlahr, M.D.

Check your pantry and refrigerator for:

• Tofu	• Celery
	• Parsley
• Turmeric	• Leaf or romaine lettuce
• Avocado	• Sprouts
• Olives	• Zuccini
• Leeks	• Carrots
• Beets	• Raisins or currants
• Pine nuts	• Orange, Limes
• Mint or basil	

7 Physical Transformers

☒ Rehydrate (EVERY DAY. Half your body weight in ounces of water)

Do at least one of the following each day:

☐ Skin Brushing

☐ Colon Cleanse

☐ Sauna Rounds

☐ Alkalinizing Bath

☐ Cleansing Bodywork

☐ Cardiovascular Sweat

Supplements & Superfoods

☒ 12–32 ounces of fresh vegetable juice. Every day.

☐ Probiotics (Acidophilus, etc)

☐ Green Drink

☐ Algae (freshwater or ocean)

☐ Enzymes

☐ Garlic clove or Allimax

☐ Colon cleansing products

BREAKFAST
Tofu Scramble .... page 125

LUNCH
Lettuce Roll Ups.. page 150
With avocado, sprouts, olives
Any sauce...page 154-162

DINNER
Zucchini & Leek Sauté (over any leftover grain)......................... page 147
Carrot & Beet Salad.. page 168
Tea

Notes & Journal: Day 8 of 28

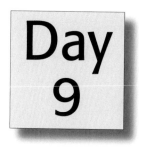

"If you think health care is expensive now, wait until you see what it costs when it's free."

P.J. O'ROURKE

Check your pantry and refrigerator for:

• Millet	• Carrots, corn, beet greens
• Quinoa	• Mushrooms, corn, arugula
• Wheat berries	• Celery, zucchini, parsley
	• Roasted red pepper
• Lentils	• Vidalia onion, salad greens
• Tofu	• Lemon
• Basil	• Sunflower seeds
• Scallions	• Olives: green and black

7 Physical Transformers

☒ Rehydrate (EVERY DAY. Half your body weight in ounces of water)

Do at least one of the following each day:

☐ Skin Brushing

☐ Colon Cleanse

☐ Sauna Rounds

☐ Alkalinizing Bath

☐ Cleansing Bodywork

☐ Cardiovascular Sweat

Supplements & Superfoods

☒ 12–32 ounces of fresh vegetable juice. Every day.

☐ Probiotics (Acidophilus, etc)

☐ Green Drink

☐ Algae (freshwater or ocean)

☐ Enzymes

☐ Garlic clove or Allimax

☐ Colon cleansing products

Breakfast

Lunch

Dinner
Tea

Notes & Journal: Day 9 of 28

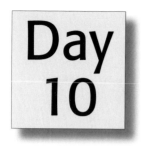

I was so inspired by your CDs that decided to do this cleanse. After suffering from psoriasis for years, I am already seeing changes. It is repairing itself from the inside out."

LORI KELLER

Check your pantry and refrigerator for:

• Barley, mochi	• Brown rice syrup
• Kale or salad greens	• Nutmeg
• Rutabagas	• Sesame oil
• Tahini	• Miso soup

7 Physical Transformers

☒ Rehydrate (EVERY DAY. Half your body weight in ounces of water)

Do at least one of the following each day:

☐ Skin Brushing

☐ Colon Cleanse

☐ Sauna Rounds

☐ Alkalinizing Bath

☐ Cleansing Bodywork

☐ Cardiovascular Sweat

Supplements & Superfoods

☒ 12–32 ounces of fresh vegetable juice. Every day.

☐ Probiotics (Acidophilus, etc)

☐ Green Drink

☐ Algae (freshwater or ocean)

☐ Enzymes

☐ Garlic clove or Allimax

☐ Colon cleansing products

Breakfast

Lunch

Dinner

Tea

Notes & Journal: Day 10 of 28

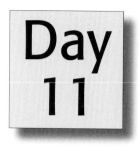

Day 11

> *"We are what we repeatedly do.
> Excellence, then, is not an act, but
> a habit."*
>
> ARISTOTLE

Check your pantry and refrigerator for:

• Rice with favorite toppings	• Carrots, celery
• Wheat berries	• Artichokes
	• Cauliflower
• Walnuts	• Apples, oranges, lemons
• Apple cider vinegar	• Mint leaves
	• Raisins
• Cannellini beans	• Capers
• Pesto	• Rosemary

7 Physical Transformers

☒ Rehydrate (EVERY DAY. Half your body weight in ounces of water)

Do at least one of the following each day:

☐ Skin Brushing

☐ Colon Cleanse

☐ Sauna Rounds

☐ Alkalinizing Bath

☐ Cleansing Bodywork

☐ Cardiovascular Sweat

Supplements & Superfoods

☒ 12–32 ounces of fresh vegetable juice. Every day.

☐ Probiotics (Acidophilus, etc)

☐ Green Drink

☐ Algae (freshwater or ocean)

☐ Enzymes

☐ Garlic clove or Allimax

☐ Colon cleansing products

BREAKFAST
Creamy Rice Cereal .... page 111

LUNCH
Wheat Berry Waldorf Salad .... page 107

DINNER
Italian Artichokes .... page 150
Roasted Vegetable & White Bean Soup with Pesto .... page 131
Tea

Notes & Journal: Day 11 of 28

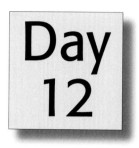

Day 12

"Why would a patient swallow a poison because he is ill, or take that which would make a well man sick."

Dr. L.F. Kebler, M.D.

Check your pantry and refrigerator for:

• Quinoa	• Kale, jicama, cauliflower
• Millet	• Green beans, celery
	• Cilantro
• Miso	• Shiitake mushrooms
• Olives	• Lime
• Pesto	• Smoothie: fresh or frozen fruit

7 Physical Transformers

☒ Rehydrate (EVERY DAY. Half your body weight in ounces of water)

Do at least one of the following each day:

☐ Skin Brushing

☐ Colon Cleanse

☐ Sauna Rounds

☐ Alkalinizing Bath

☐ Cleansing Bodywork

☐ Cardiovascular Sweat

Supplements & Superfoods

☒ 12–32 ounces of fresh vegetable juice. Every day.

☐ Probiotics (Acidophilus, etc)

☐ Green Drink

☐ Algae (freshwater or ocean)

☐ Enzymes

☐ Garlic clove or Allimax

☐ Colon cleansing products

Breakfast

Lunch

Dinner
Tea

Notes & Journal: Day 12 of 28

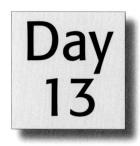

Day 13

"After a LOT of detoxing, my 68-year old husband is finally off all medication. He feels better than he has in years. Cleansing is now a permanent part of our lifestyle."

MARY SOYENOVA

Check your pantry and refrigerator for:

• Mochi	• Avocado, burdock, squash
• Chickpeas	• Carrots, celery, cucumber
• Almonds	• Sweet potatoes, potatoes
• Kuzu powder	• Mushrooms, peas, parsnips
• Beans	• Basil, sage, thyme, oregano

7 Physical Transformers

☒ Rehydrate (EVERY DAY. Half your body weight in ounces of water)

Do at least one of the following each day:

☐ Skin Brushing

☐ Colon Cleanse

☐ Sauna Rounds

☐ Alkalinizing Bath

☐ Cleansing Bodywork

☐ Cardiovascular Sweat

Supplements & Superfoods

☒ 12–32 ounces of fresh vegetable juice. Every day.

☐ Probiotics (Acidophilus, etc)

☐ Green Drink

☐ Algae (freshwater or ocean)

☐ Enzymes

☐ Garlic clove or Allimax

☐ Colon cleansing products

BREAKFAST

LUNCH

Raw vegetables

DINNER

Tea

Notes & Journal: Day 13 of 28

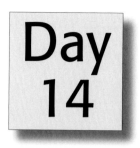

Day 14

"*Every drug increases and compli-cates the patients condition.*"

Dr. Robert Henderson, M.D.

Check your pantry and refrigerator for:

• Rice	• Kale, red onion
• Wild salmon	• Bok choy, celeriac, potatoes
• Kombu	• Capers, basil
• Arame	
• Powdered wasabi	• Sauerkraut
• Olives	• Sesame Seeds
• Cranberries	• Cardomom

7 Physical Transformers

☒ Rehydrate (EVERY DAY. Half your body weight in ounces of water)

Do at least one of the following each day:

☐ Skin Brushing

☐ Colon Cleanse

☐ Sauna Rounds

☐ Alkalinizing Bath

☐ Cleansing Bodywork

☐ Cardiovascular Sweat

Supplements & Superfoods

☒ 12–32 ounces of fresh vegetable juice. Every day.

☐ Probiotics (Acidophilus, etc)

☐ Green Drink

☐ Algae (freshwater or ocean)

☐ Enzymes

☐ Garlic clove or Allimax

☐ Colon cleansing products

BREAKFAST

LUNCH

DINNER
Tea

Notes & Journal: Day 14 of 28

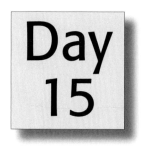

"Every educated physician knows that most diseases are not appreciably helped by medicine."

Dr. Richard C. Cabot, M.D. 1998,
Mass. Gen. Hospital

Check your pantry and refrigerator for:

• Essene bread	• Avocado, cucumber
• Rice	• Parsley, shallots
	• Acorn squash
• Pomegranate	• Basil, capers, mushrooms
• Lemon, lime, banana	• Frozen or fresh peas

7 Physical Transformers

☒ Rehydrate (EVERY DAY. Half your body weight in ounces of water)

Do at least one of the following each day:

☐ Skin Brushing

☐ Colon Cleanse

☐ Sauna Rounds

☐ Alkalinizing Bath

☐ Cleansing Bodywork

☐ Cardiovascular Sweat

Supplements & Superfoods

☒ 12–32 ounces of fresh vegetable juice. Every day.

☐ Probiotics (Acidophilus, etc)

☐ Green Drink

☐ Algae (freshwater or ocean)

☐ Enzymes

☐ Garlic clove or Allimax

☐ Colon cleansing products

BREAKFAST
Essene bread toasted with coconut oil

LUNCH
Leftover Grain Bowl .... page 116
(such as Avocado, Cucumber, with Arame Tapenade over rice with olive oil and lemon dressing... basically, this is a clean-out-the-refrigerator day)

DINNER
Slow Cooker Mushroom Risotto with Peas .... page 108
Maple Roasted Acorn Squash .... page 145
Pomegranate Salad .... page 171
Tea

Notes & Journal: Day 15 of 28

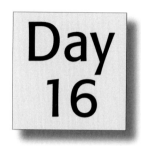

"My skin has been extremely dry for many years; it literally would bleed on a daily basis. I am happy to report that after just a month of cleansing, it is now normal, for the first time in decades. Bravo Scott."

SARAH SMITH

Check your pantry and refrigerator for:

• Teff	• Salad greens
• Rice	• Carrots, beets
• Cashews, other nuts	• Parsnips, onions
• Miso soup	• Almonds

7 Physical Transformers

☒ Rehydrate (EVERY DAY. Half your body weight in ounces of water)

Do at least one of the following each day:

☐ Skin Brushing

☐ Colon Cleanse

☐ Sauna Rounds

☐ Alkalinizing Bath

☐ Cleansing Bodywork

☐ Cardiovascular Sweat

Supplements & Superfoods

☒ 12–32 ounces of fresh vegetable juice. Every day.

☐ Probiotics (Acidophilus, etc)

☐ Green Drink

☐ Algae (freshwater or ocean)

☐ Enzymes

☐ Garlic clove or Allimax

☐ Colon cleansing products

BREAKFAST
Teff Porridge .... page 104

Roasted tamari nuts .... page 175

LUNCH
Green Salad (try arugula, frissee and orange salad)

Miso Soup.. page 127

DINNER
Roasted Root Vegetables .... page 149

Brown Rice .... page 103

Cashew Miso Dressing.. page 157

Tea

Notes & Journal: Day 16 of 28

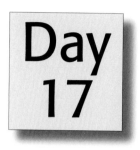

Day 17

"Medicines are of subordinate importance because of their very nature they can only work symptomatically."

DR. HANS KUSCHE, M.D.

Check your pantry and refrigerator for:

• Almond butter	• Cabbage, carrots, scallions
• Umeboshi vinegar	• Bok choy, fresh dill
• Tofu	• Cucumbers
• Brown rice syrup	• Lemon
• Red aduki beans	• Hijiki, nori seaweed
	• Sunflower seeds

7 Physical Transformers

☒ Rehydrate (EVERY DAY. Half your body weight in ounces of water)

Do at least one of the following each day:

☐ Skin Brushing

☐ Colon Cleanse

☐ Sauna Rounds

☐ Alkalinizing Bath

☐ Cleansing Bodywork

☐ Cardiovascular Sweat

Supplements & Superfoods

☒ 12–32 ounces of fresh vegetable juice. Every day.

☐ Probiotics (Acidophilus, etc)

☐ Green Drink

☐ Algae (freshwater or ocean)

☐ Enzymes

☐ Garlic clove or Allimax

☐ Colon cleansing products

BREAKFAST
Fried grain (left over grain with vegetables)

LUNCH
Asian Sesame Coleslaw .... page 167
Tofu Quick Bake.. page 124

DINNER
Grain Bowl .... page 116
Combine Red aduki beans, bok choy, nori, sunflower seeds, over rice with cashew miso sauce
Sweet and Sour Cucumbers.. page 169

Notes & Journal: Day 17 of 28

218

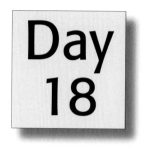

Day 18

"Be so strong that nothing can disturb your peace of mind. Talk health, talk happiness, and talk prosperity. Be too big for worry."

CHRISTIAN D. LARSEN

Check your pantry and refrigerator for:

• Potatoes	• Cilantro, jalepenos
• Kimchi	• Alfalfa sprouts, kale
• Aduki bean sprouts	• Avocado, leeks, carrots
• Cashews	• Lettuce or cabbage leaves
• Fruit, fresh or frozen	

7 Physical Transformers

☒ Rehydrate (EVERY DAY. Half your body weight in ounces of water)

Do at least one of the following each day:

☐ Skin Brushing

☐ Colon Cleanse

☐ Sauna Rounds

☐ Alkalinizing Bath

☐ Cleansing Bodywork

☐ Cardiovascular Sweat

Supplements & Superfoods

☒ 12–32 ounces of fresh vegetable juice. Every day.

☐ Probiotics (Acidophilus, etc)

☐ Green Drink

☐ Algae (freshwater or ocean)

☐ Enzymes

☐ Garlic clove or Allimax

☐ Colon cleansing products

Breakfast

Lunch

Dinner

Tea

Notes & Journal: Day 18 of 28

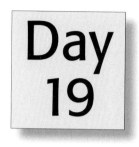

"To love what you do, and feel that it matters—how could anything be more fun?"

ANONYMOUS

Check your pantry and refrigerator for:

• Essene bread	• Carrots, cucumbers, sprouts
• Wheat berries	• Scallions, collard greens
• Quinoa	• Cilantro, lemon grass
• Tofu	• Mint, Cumin seeds
• Almonds	• Mung sprouts
	• Lemon, lime
• Coconut milk	• Fresh chili pepper
• Pumpkin seeds	• Jalapeno

7 Physical Transformers

☒ Rehydrate (EVERY DAY. Half your body weight in ounces of water)

Do at least one of the following each day:

☐ Skin Brushing

☐ Colon Cleanse

☐ Sauna Rounds

☐ Alkalinizing Bath

☐ Cleansing Bodywork

☐ Cardiovascular Sweat

Supplements & Superfoods

☒ 12–32 ounces of fresh vegetable juice. Every day.

☐ Probiotics (Acidophilus, etc)

☐ Green Drink

☐ Algae (freshwater or ocean)

☐ Enzymes

☐ Garlic clove or Allimax

☐ Colon cleansing products

Breakfast
Baked Tofu.. page 124

Toasted Essene bread with coconut oil

Lunch
Collard Rollups .... page 150

With wheat berries, cucumber, and carrot (or anything you want)

Almond Hummus.. page 120

Dinner
Spicy Thai Soup with Coconut Milk................................. page 129

Quinoa.. page 102

Tea

Notes & Journal: Day 19 of 28

222

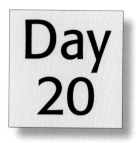

Day 20

"Who's script are you running? Who taught you what you believe? Why do you believe it? Are you sure it's true? Are you aware of the impact it has?"

ANONYMOUS

Check your pantry and refrigerator for:

• Essene bread	• Celery, romaine lettuce
• Barley	• Arugula, scallions, parsley
• Cannellini or white beans	• Basil, capers
	• Red onion
• Olives	• Portobello mushrooms
• Orange, lemons, limes	• Mint or sage
• Grapefruit, cranberries	

7 Physical Transformers

[x] Rehydrate (EVERY DAY. Half your body weight in ounces of water)

Do at least one of the following each day:

[ ] Skin Brushing

[ ] Colon Cleanse

[ ] Sauna Rounds

[ ] Alkalinizing Bath

[ ] Cleansing Bodywork

[ ] Cardiovascular Sweat

Supplements & Superfoods

[x] 12–32 ounces of fresh vegetable juice. Every day.

[ ] Probiotics (Acidophilus, etc)

[ ] Green Drink

[ ] Algae (freshwater or ocean)

[ ] Enzymes

[ ] Garlic clove or Allimax

[ ] Colon cleansing products

Breakfast
Cranberry grapefruit compote .... page 174

with Essene bread

Lunch
Tuscan Bean and Vegetable Salad .... page 121

Dinner
Marinated Portobellos with Barley Pilaf..110

Serve over raw arugula

Tea

Notes & Journal: Day 20 of 28

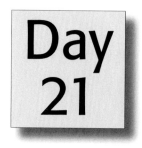

Day 21

"The cause of most disease is in the poisonous drugs physician superstitiously give in order to effect a cure."

Dr. Charles E. Page, M.D.

Check your pantry and refrigerator for:

• Mochi	• Sea palm
• Rice	• Umeboshi vinegar
• Fresh cod	• Rapini or other greens
• Olives	• Jicama
• MIso Soup	

7 Physical Transformers

☒ Rehydrate (EVERY DAY. Half your body weight in ounces of water)

Do at least one of the following each day:

☐ Skin Brushing

☐ Colon Cleanse

☐ Sauna Rounds

☐ Alkalinizing Bath

☐ Cleansing Bodywork

☐ Cardiovascular Sweat

Supplements & Superfoods

☒ 12–32 ounces of fresh vegetable juice. Every day.

☐ Probiotics (Acidophilus, etc)

☐ Green Drink

☐ Algae (freshwater or ocean)

☐ Enzymes

☐ Garlic clove or Allimax

☐ Colon cleansing products

Breakfast
Baked mochi.. page 50

Lunch
Sea Palm, Weed of Darkness... page 144
Grain Bowl .... page 116

Dinner
Cod with Rapini, Garlic and Olives .... page 152
Rice .... page 103
Miso Soup (or some variation) .... page 127
Tea

Notes & Journal: Day 21 of 28

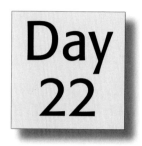

Day 22

"It's supposed to be a secret, but I'll tell you anyway. We doctors do nothing. We only help and encourage the doctor within."

DR. ALBERT SCHWEITZER, M.D.

Check your pantry and refrigerator for:

• Rice	• Napa cabbage, scallions
• Tofu	• Sweet potato, kale
• Rice vinegar	• Red onion, cilantro
• Brown rice Syrup	• Basil, avocado, capers
• Peanuts, sunflower seeds	• Carrots, cabbage, sprouts
• Kalamata olives	• Snow pea pods
• Lime	• Arame

7 Physical Transformers

☒ Rehydrate (EVERY DAY. Half your body weight in ounces of water)

Do at least one of the following each day:

☐ Skin Brushing

☐ Colon Cleanse

☐ Sauna Rounds

☐ Alkalinizing Bath

☐ Cleansing Bodywork

☐ Cardiovascular Sweat

Supplements & Superfoods

☒ 12–32 ounces of fresh vegetable juice. Every day.

☐ Probiotics (Acidophilus, etc)

☐ Green Drink

☐ Algae (freshwater or ocean)

☐ Enzymes

☐ Garlic clove or Allimax

☐ Colon cleansing products

Breakfast

Lunch

Salad (try avocado, sunflower sprouts, arame tapenade, olive oil, lemon)

Dinner

Steamed or Boiled Kale

Tea

Notes & Journal: Day 22 of 28

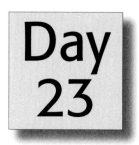

Day 23

The only rule is to work. If you work, it will lead to something. It's the people who do all of the work all the time who eventually catch on to things."

SISTER CORITA KENT

Check your pantry and refrigerator for:

• Oat groats	• Kale, red onion
• Rice	• Carrots,
• Chickpeas	• Red onion, cucumbers
• Tofu	• Mint, avocado
	• Purslane, napa cabbage
• Nori	• Scallions
• Pickled ginger	
• Pine nuts	• Orange, lemon
• Wasabi powder	• Almonds

7 Physical Transformers

☒ Rehydrate (EVERY DAY. Half your body weight in ounces of water)

Do at least one of the following each day:

☐ Skin Brushing

☐ Colon Cleanse

☐ Sauna Rounds

☐ Alkalinizing Bath

☐ Cleansing Bodywork

☐ Cardiovascular Sweat

Supplements & Superfoods

☒ 12–32 ounces of fresh vegetable juice. Every day.

☐ Probiotics (Acidophilus, etc)

☐ Green Drink

☐ Algae (freshwater or ocean)

☐ Enzymes

☐ Garlic clove or Allimax

☐ Colon cleansing products

BREAKFAST

LUNCH

DINNER

Tea

Notes & Journal: Day 23 of 28

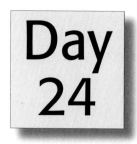

Day 24

"What is necessary to change a person is to change his awareness of himself."

ABRAHAM H. MASLOW

Check your pantry and refrigerator for:

• Essene bread	• Dandelion or endive
• Fava beans	• Peas, Jerusalem Artichokes
• Capers, thyme	• Parsley, carrots, celery
• Lentils	• Shiitake mushrooms
• Miso	• Escarole or endive

7 Physical Transformers

☒ Rehydrate (EVERY DAY. Half your body weight in ounces of water)

Do at least one of the following each day:

☐ Skin Brushing

☐ Colon Cleanse

☐ Sauna Rounds

☐ Alkalinizing Bath

☐ Cleansing Bodywork

☐ Cardiovascular Sweat

Supplements & Superfoods

☒ 12–32 ounces of fresh vegetable juice. Every day.

☐ Probiotics (Acidophilus, etc)

☐ Green Drink

☐ Algae (freshwater or ocean)

☐ Enzymes

☐ Garlic clove or Allimax

☐ Colon cleansing products

BREAKFAST
Miso Soup.. page 127

Essene Bread

LUNCH
Dandelion salad

Savory Fava Beans with Capers, Garlic & Thyme.......................... page 118

DINNER
Jerusalem Artichoke, Peas & Shiitake Mushrooms....................... page 138

Lentil & Escarole Soup.. page 131

Tea

Notes & Journal:

Day 24 of 28

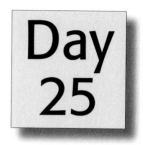

Day
25

"I've known Scott Ohlgren for 15 years. He consistently lives his vision of health. I heartily endorse his system of wellness."

DR. DALE MABE,
FAMILY MEDICINE PHYSICIAN

Check your pantry and refrigerator for:

• Buckwheat groats	• Carrots, parsley, turnips
• Rice	• Collard or another hearty green
• Almonds	• Potatoes, burdock root
• Raw honey	• Pineapple, apples
• Sunflower seeds	• Pomegrante, lime, lemons
	• Papaya or mango, banana

7 Physical Transformers

☒ Rehydrate (EVERY DAY. Half your body weight in ounces of water)

Do at least one of the following each day:

☐ Skin Brushing

☐ Colon Cleanse

☐ Sauna Rounds

☐ Alkalinizing Bath

☐ Cleansing Bodywork

☐ Cardiovascular Sweat

Supplements & Superfoods

☒ 12–32 ounces of fresh vegetable juice. Every day.

☐ Probiotics (Acidophilus, etc)

☐ Green Drink

☐ Algae (freshwater or ocean)

☐ Enzymes

☐ Garlic clove or Allimax

☐ Colon cleansing products

Breakfast

Lunch

Dinner

Tea

Notes & Journal: Day 25 of 28

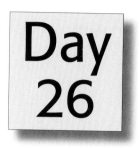

"Be kind, for everyone you meet is fighting a hard battle."

PLATO

Check your pantry and refrigerator for:

• Kamut	• Carrot
• Barley	• Jicama
• Quinoa	• Winter squash
• Chickpeas	• Cucumber
• Tahini	• Sage, thyme
• Coconut Milk (optional)	• Apple, dried fruits
• Sunflower seeds	• Vanilla extract

7 Physical Transformers

[X] Rehydrate (EVERY DAY. Half your body weight in ounces of water)

Do at least one of the following each day:

[ ] Skin Brushing

[ ] Colon Cleanse

[ ] Sauna Rounds

[ ] Alkalinizing Bath

[ ] Cleansing Bodywork

[ ] Cardiovascular Sweat

Supplements & Superfoods

[X] 12–32 ounces of fresh vegetable juice. Every day.

[ ] Probiotics (Acidophilus, etc)

[ ] Green Drink

[ ] Algae (freshwater or ocean)

[ ] Enzymes

[ ] Garlic clove or Allimax

[ ] Colon cleansing products

Breakfast

Lunch

Dinner
Tea

Notes & Journal: Day 26 of 28

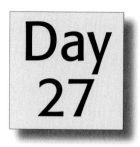

Day 27

"After all the trouble you go to, you get about as much actual food out of eating an artichoke as you would from licking 30 or 40 postage stamps."

Miss Piggy

Check your pantry and refrigerator for:

• Essene bread	• Carrot, parsley, cilantro
• Seitan	• Acorn squash
• Tofu	• Scallions, napa cabbage
• Tempeh	• Bay leaves, oregano
• Dashi	• Chili peppers
• Anise seeds	• Cinnamon sticks, oregano
• Brown rice vinegar	• Lemon

7 Physical Transformers

☒ Rehydrate (EVERY DAY. Half your body weight in ounces of water)

Do at least one of the following each day:

☐ Skin Brushing

☐ Colon Cleanse

☐ Sauna Rounds

☐ Alkalinizing Bath

☐ Cleansing Bodywork

☐ Cardiovascular Sweat

Supplements & Superfoods

☒ 12–32 ounces of fresh vegetable juice. Every day.

☐ Probiotics (Acidophilus, etc)

☐ Green Drink

☐ Algae (freshwater or ocean)

☐ Enzymes

☐ Garlic clove or Allimax

☐ Colon cleansing products

BREAKFAST
Tofu scramble .... page 125

Essene bread

LUNCH
Tempeh Chimi Churri .... page 124

Steamed vegetables (anything) with dressing

DINNER
Roasted Salt & Pepper Squash .... page 146

Asian Seitan Soup with Cinnamon .... page 136

Tea

Notes & Journal:
Day 27 of 28

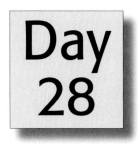

Day 28

I did my first full 28-day cleanse in May. It felt like I had treated myself to a month at a very good spa. I am planning my second cleanse this January.

CAROLYN GUTHLEBEN

Check your pantry and refrigerator for:

• Smoothie or fresh fruit	• Avocado, scallions
• Rice	• Green beans, cilantro
• Tempeh	• Jalapeno
• Black beans	• Lemon, limes, mango
• Cashews	• Coconut milk

7 Physical Transformers

☒ Rehydrate (EVERY DAY. Half your body weight in ounces of water)

Do at least one of the following each day:

☐ Skin Brushing

☐ Colon Cleanse

☐ Sauna Rounds

☐ Alkalinizing Bath

☐ Cleansing Bodywork

☐ Cardiovascular Sweat

Supplements & Superfoods

☒ 12–32 ounces of fresh vegetable juice. Every day.

☐ Probiotics (Acidophilus, etc)

☐ Green Drink

☐ Algae (freshwater or ocean)

☐ Enzymes

☐ Garlic clove or Allimax

☐ Colon cleansing products

Breakfast

Lunch

Dinner

Tea

Notes & Journal: Day 28 of 28

Sources Section

So many of the items mentioned throughout this book can now be found in any large health food store. Still, there are a few hard-to-find items that are so important to a cleansing lifestyle, especially those items that are better to buy in bulk (I buy kilos of salt, not small packages); or, in the case of fermented foods, difficult to find unpasteurized. Here are some sources.

Superfoods

Celtic Gray Sea salt.................... 1800 TOP SALT www.Celtic-Seasalt.com

Kitchenware

Pressure cookers, etc. .... www.HowHealthWorks.com

Sea Fresh Water Algae Companies

Maine Coast Sea Vegetable ....www.SeaVeg.com

Mendocino Sea Vegetable .... www.SeaWeed.net

Rising Tide ....www.loveSeaWeed.com

Ocean Harvest...www.ohsv.net

Wild Bluegreen Algae...www.CellTech.com

Naturally Fermented Food Companies

Real Pickles ....www.RealPickles.com

Bubbies ....www.Bubbies.com

Rejuvenative Company ....www.Rejunevative.com

Miso (unpasteurized) ....

Umeboshi products

South River Miso Company .... www.SouthRiverMiso.com

Herbal Formulas

Dancing Willow Herbs .... www.DancingWillowHerbs.com

Cleansing Health Practitioners

Dr. Nasha Winters .... www.NamasteHealthCenter.com

Russell Mariani...www.HealthEquest.com

Virginia Harper (live-in cleansing program) ....wwwKiOfLife.com

For large list of cleansing practitioners......... www.HowHealthWorks.com

ABOUT SCOTT OHLGREN

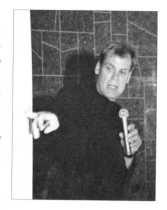

Scott Ohlgren is an enthusiastic student, teacher, beneficiary, and author of the natural healing paradigm. Raised in Wisconsin, where Spam and Velveeta cheese were considered part of the four Food Groups, his introduction to the diet-symptom, diet-health connection came just in time. At age 19, tired of acne, sinus problems and tetracycline, a friend shoved a book into his hands, saying, "Change your diet, and those symptoms will go away." Five weeks later, these symptoms were gone.

Since then, periodic cellular cleansing has been a central part of his life and is the main reason why he hasn't used a single antibiotic or prescription drug since 1976. He is a 1985 Kushi Institute graduate, a nine-month intensive live-and-study program on food sciences. He studied at the two-year Rolfing Institute and became certified as a Rolfing Practitioner in 1988. He has sold over 90,000 tapes, videos and books on the diet/disease, diet/health connection, and he has been featured in the Bay Area Monthly and Success Magazine. Scott's been the keynote speaker at the International Association of Colon Hydrotherapy annual meeting. He is board-certified by the American Association of Drugless Practitioners as a Holistic Health Practitioner, and is accredited by the Florida International University for CEU credits. Since 2001, his online 28-day Cleansing Program has taken over 12,000 participants through the same process that he learned 30 years ago.

Scott has become an outspoken proponent, lecturer, and author for a drug, pain and disease-free life, using real food nutrition as one's main medicine cabinet. And he thinks America's "health-care crisis" is a bunch of hooey, the obvious outcome of a culture that has forgotten how to feed itself.

He lives in Boulder, CO, with his wife, Gael.

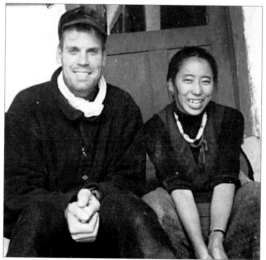

Scott in Nepal, with Nepalese cook

ABOUT JOANN TOMASULO

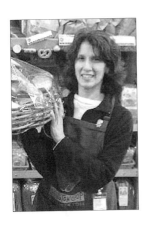

With roots steeped in the tradition of home-cooked meals, Joann Tomasulo has a passion for good food. At eleven years of age, her first job was in her Italian grandparents' food store in downtown Buffalo, New York, cleaning heads of lettuce and shining apples. When her mom went back to work, cooking became mandatory for all family members.

In her twenties, Joann found herself prone to crabbiness and depression. After her fiancé handed her a book on cleansing and colon care, she realized that the cause of her ailments had been due to the gradual increase of processed foods in her diet. She incorporated more whole foods into her life and turned her health around. This shift in understanding the connection between food and health launched her passion for the art of healthy cooking.

By combining her 25 years of knowledge of whole food nutrition with traditional down-home cooking, Joann has developed these healthy and delicious recipes for the 28-Day Cleanse.

Even with her extremely busy schedule as a Marketing Manager of the local food cooperative, Joann still loves to spend time feeding her lucky friends and family nutritious, wholesome meals; many of which she shares with us in this book. Preparing meals continues to be a combination of creativity, health and practicality. She loves the challenge of sharing food with others that is unexpected, simple and delicious.

She currently lives in Buffalo, New York, with her husband, Gary (still grateful for handing her that book), and son, Finn.

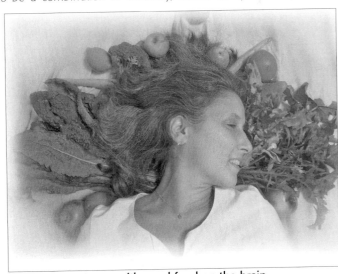

Joann with good food on the brain

MEDICAL DISCLAIMER

If you were born in—or currently reside in—America, it is important that you read the following medical disclaimer. Strangely, all other countries are exempt.

It is always best to consult a physician/prescription drug provider before undertaking any major shift in your diet.

The information given in this book is nothing more than opinions or suggestions, and is therefore protected under the First Amendment of the United States Constitution, which grants the right to discuss openly and freely all matters and viewpoints. If that last sentence does not make sense, or makes you want to sue someone, please consult your physician/prescription drug provider.

These viewpoints found herein should not be used for the diagnosis or treatment of any ailment. Nothing said, or hinted at being said, or imagined being said, or told by a psychic that the author said, should be construed as medical advice.

None of the writers of these viewpoints can guarantee the accuracy or completeness of any information conveyed. The absence of a warning for a given recipe, vitamin, mineral, herb, plant, street drug, diet soda, Swanson's Frozen Dinner, or any combination of these substances should not be construed to indicate that the substance combination is safe, appropriate or effective for any given consumer. In particular, in no event will NaviQuest Corporation, How Health Works™, Scott Ohlgren, family members both living and dead, or ex-girlfriends (Scott) or boyfriends (Joann) going back as far as 1972 be liable for direct, indirect, special, incidental, secondary, or consequential damages resulting from any application of these viewpoints, even if advised that the viewpoints are good for you (examples of advice: "Eat this..." "We suggest..." "The sky is falling..."). If you have questions about your health care or another person's health care, please consult your physician/prescription drug provider.

All of the information contained within this book, as well as suggested websites, audio and other written material is provided with the understanding that the information and its providers shall not be responsible to any person or entity for any loss or damage caused, or alleged to have been caused, directly or indirectly by or from the information, ideas, or suggestions. Your participation with any of these ideas or edible items is solely done so at your own risk. If the concept of "your own risk" and "personal responsibility" is not fully grasped, understood, and practiced in daily life, the writers of this material request that you close this book, put it down, and not utilize any of the suggestions. Instead, please consult your physician/prescription drug provider.

Furthermore, if you are currently taking any medications whatsoever (prescription or over-the-counter), being medically supervised for the care and treatment of any illness (especially taking chemicals for chemical depression), scheduled for surgery, taking immune-suppressant drugs, or simply not sure what to do, please consult your physician/prescription drug provider.

The suggestions and opinions set forth are nothing but opinions, and should not be interpreted as anything but opinions. The entire risk as to the results and performance of these opinions are assumed by you. If the instructions are defective, you, and not the authors, assume the entire cost of all necessary servicing, repair or correction.

This book contains no MSG, GMO seed stock, or other artificial ingredients.

No animals were harmed in the creation of this book.

Contents of this book may be hot. Point away from face when opening. Do not plug into an outlet near an open body of water or bathtub.

Keep out of reach of children.

Do not induce vomiting.

Objects in mirror may be closer than they appear.

If you are pregnant or nursing... congratulations.

INDEX

B

C

D

E

F

G

T

U

Udo Erasmus 58

Umeboshi 63, 65

Unsaturated 58

Ulcerative Colitis 10

Unpasteurized cultured foods 62

Uremia 20

V

Vegan 28

Vegetable Oils, to avoid 60

Vegetable Stock 128

Velveeta cheese 12

Visceral manipulation 36

Vomiting 20, 78

Vegetable Dishes 138

Vegetables 54

Vegetarianism 28

Virginia Harper 241

Vitamin Cottage 26

W

Wakame 66, 67

Walnut 175

Water Cure Drink 178

Waukesha 12

Weight gain 5

Weston Price 13

Wheat Berries, basic recipe 104

Wheatgrass 93

Whitaker i

Wild Oats 26

William Campbell Douglass 59

Wisconsin 12

Waldorf Salad 107

Watercress 55

Water retention 66

Weight control 76

Westbrae 52

Wheat 101, 104

Wheat Berry 107

Wheatgrass 40

Whole Foods 26

Wild Rice, basic recipe 104

William Osler 16

Y

Yeast 14, 19

Yogurt 32

Z

Zinc 66

ORDER FORM

Item #1. *Cellular Cleansing Made Easy* (the book) $15
Item #2. *Real Food, Real Health* (the 3-CD audiobook)................. $40
Item #3. *The 28-Day Cleansing Program* (this book) $28

Item #4. All three items above (30% off).. $59

Name: _____

Address: _____

City: _____

State: _____ ZIP: _____

Telephone: _____

Email: _____

Visa/MC: _____

Name on card: _____ Expires: _____

Item # _____ x _____ = $_____

Item # _____ x _____ = $_____

Item # _____ x _____ = $_____

Shipping: $6.00 flat fee, regardless of order size $ _____

Total of this order: $ _____

Fax orders: 303 527-0270
Email orders: sales@howhealthworks.com
Postal orders: 7440 N. 49th St, Longmont, CO 80503-8847